As Thin as You Think

Discover the Keys to Unlocking Your Weight Loss Power

To my amazing friend, Roslyn -
Peace, joy, health & happiness
Kristin Volk Funk

Also by Kristin Volk Funk, M.Ed., CCH

Available Recordings

Weight Loss

Quit Smoking

Stress Release

End Insomnia

Relaxation Techniques

Self-Esteem and Confidence

Healing and Pain Control

Sports Performance

Successful Parenting

Enhanced Learning

Enhanced Memory

Healing from Loss

Inner Peace

All of the above may be ordered by visiting:
www.newhealthvisions.com

As Thin as You Think

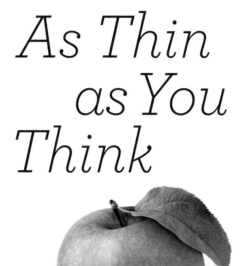

*Discover the Keys to Unlocking
Your Weight Loss Power*

KRISTIN VOLK FUNK, M.Ed., CCH

BEAVER'S POND PRESS

ISBN 13: 978-1-59298-417-6

Library of Congress Catalog Number: 2011931208
Printed in the United States of America
First Printing: 2012
15   14   13   12   11   5   4   3   2   1

Cover and interior design by Carol Logie

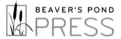

BEAVER'S POND
PRESS

Beaver's Pond Press, Inc.
7104 Ohms Lane, Suite 101
Edina, MN 55439-2129
(952) 829-8818
www.BeaversPondPress.com

To order, visit www.BookHouseFulfillment.com
www.BeaversPondBooks.com
or call 1-800-901-3480. Reseller discounts available.

Disclaimer

*The ideas presented in this publication are intended for educational purposes only and are not intended
to take the place of medical or psychological advice from a trained medical professional. This publication is sold with the understanding that the author is not dispensing medical, health, psychological, or
any other kind of personal professional services. Readers are advised to consult a physician or other
qualified health professionals before adopting any of the ideas in this book.*

*The author specifically disclaims all responsibility for any liability, loss, or risk, personal or
otherwise, which is incurred as a consequence, directly or indirectly, of the use and application of
any of the contents of this book.*

*With the exception of the testimonials, names of persons mentioned in this book have been
changed to protect their identity.*

For my sons, Bernard and Joseph—
you have brought so much joy to my life.
I love you dearly.

Praise for Kristin Volk Funk's Work and
the **As Thin As You Think** *Program:*

When I first started Kristin's program, I weighed 220 pounds. With her techniques, I easily lost 40 pounds and have stayed at a healthy 180 pounds for over two years. Kristin got me past the psychological walls that used to keep me overweight. I quit smoking thanks to Kristin as well! —BRIAN DUNGAN, CHANHASSEN, MINNESOTA

With Kristin's program, I have lost a total of 86 pounds so far, and I am only 17 pounds from my original goal! I feel fantastic, and it has been really fun shopping for my upcoming vacation!

—CINDY STUNEK, BAXTER, MINNESOTA

Kristin's As Thin As You Think *seminar gave me the focus to lose and keep off 18 pounds. The class empowered me to exchange chocolate and bread cravings with a strong desire for vegetables and other healthy food.* —DEE CANTALICE, MILLSTONE TOWNSHIP, NEW JERSEY

With Kristin's help I lost 25 pounds without exercise and have effortlessly kept the weight off. The hypnosis was great. It took away the cravings for fast food and candy, and I was rarely hungry. Now my refrigerator is filled with vegetables, and junk food no longer tempts me. —JIM CLAFFEY, MAHTOMEDI, MINNESOTA

I lost 9 pounds the first week of my program with Kristin. I was never able to diet for more than a week before, and now I have no desire for the pizza, cheese, and pop that are around the house. What I love about Kristin's program is that I don't think about food between meals or at night. It's the easiest thing ever. I can't emphasize enough how simple it is. Kristin's techniques are amazing!

—LIZ DICKINSON, CANNON FALLS, MINNESOTA

Since my weight loss program with Kristin began last week, I'm drinking tons of water, keeping a food journal, and listening to the CD. I have also worked out twice at the gym. I am calm, committed, and happy. —STEVE BRIGGS, GRANTSBURG, WISCONSIN

Thanks to Kristin, I was able to let go of my emotional addiction to food and lost 25 pounds. I'm in control again!
—KAREN RAJTAR, HAM LAKE, MINNESOTA

My experience with Kristin has been nothing but positive. Her combination of nutritional counseling and hypnotherapy has made losing a lifetime of poor eating habits and excess weight very easy. The weight is melting off of me! The program is about switching bad lifestyle habits for healthy ones, and it is not difficult. I don't know why I waited so long to do this.
—SUE SMART, HAM LAKE, MINNESOTA

With Kristin's techniques and advice, I now have no desire for pop. I now crave vegetables! I just did what she told me to do, and the hypnosis made it easy. I feel wonderful. I don't even notice the vending machine and junk food that's in the office every day. And my mid-afternoon slump is totally gone. I have so much energy all day long. Eating healthy is a lot of fun now. I am having fun at this!
—MONA KLAREN, COTTAGE GROVE, MINNESOTA

Kristin's book was a real eye-opener for me! For the first time ever, I was able to connect past weight gain with specific physical or emotional events – and even better, I've been able to release those emotions and detach from the events totally. Proof that this works is that I lost eight pounds in three weeks by making just three changes in my normal routine.
—MARY STOFFEL, Author of The Practical Power of Shamanism: Heal Your Life, Loves and Losses.

TABLE OF CONTENTS

PART I: Letting Go of Emotional Eating

PART II: Developing Your Personal Weight Loss Plan

If you are overweight, you are not to blame! It is not your fault!

In the past decade, we have been saturated with dieting information. We all know that sugar, transfats, and lack of exercise are bad for us. With all of the information available, why is obesity growing at alarming rates? Why are we feeling such frustration and guilt as we lose weight only to gain it again?

This is not a diet book. It is a book that will allow you to feel the confidence, self-love, and motivation to turn away from the thoughts and feelings that cause you to gain weight. This is a book to help you take charge of your mind.

When you change on the inside, the reflection you see in the mirror changes.

Before you change your relationship to food, you must first change your relationship with yourself. Traditional diets are about looking at the outside world: what you buy at the grocery store, what gym to join, the numbers on the scale. As long as you keep your focus on the outside, you will go on and then off the diet. You will lose and then gain the weight. If nothing on the inside (your heart and mind) changes, you will stay stuck on the failure plan of diets.

This book is an invitation to walk on the Success Path that will lead you to happy, healthy, and, most importantly, permanent weight loss.

This book helps you to lovingly address the cause of your weight problems. It is not just about what foods to eat and how to exercise, but also about what you have innocently internalized in your heart and mind. With gentleness, this book will help you heal the unconscious, mistaken beliefs that have led you to overeat.

When you change the Inner You into a healthier one, you will start to view food differently.

This profound change does not require a lot of time or money. If you're like most people today, you have already made the costly investment of both and have been devastated to find the weight creep back up again.

The profound change to permanent weight loss simply requires a small willingness to begin the journey.

Take one small step—see and feel the positive results. Take another small step ... and another ... with each small step you feel more hopeful. You begin to turn your attention away from food and feelings of failure and to say "no" to cravings. You begin to walk with self-control and embrace the change that is yours to make. Before you know it, you are permanently walking a path of health as a slender, self-loving person.

This book is about a permanent healing not just in your relationship with food, but more importantly in your relationship to yourself. This book will give you the keys.

May we begin?

After earning my master's degree, finishing my internship, and working several years as a counselor, I became intrigued with the clinical applications of hypnosis. I decided to visit several local hypnotherapists to personally experience the healing powers of hypnosis and to become familiar with the various techniques. Along the way, I was fortunate to meet my mentor, Geri Rudd, who was in the process of slowly retiring from private practice.

Geri was a member of MENSA and had a master's of social work degree. She was brilliant, kind, and insightful, and to my great fortune, she took me under her wing. I began a fast track apprenticeship program with her, with the understanding that I would assume her practice when she retired. This was an exciting time for me, as I knew I had found a truly effective technique that would help people achieve their health goals. I've been hooked on hypnotherapy ever since.

After practicing hypnosis under the tutelage of Geri, I was ready for my first solo sessions.

My first client was a long-time smoker who wanted to quit the smoking habit because it was ruining his health. This middle-aged man, who had smoked two packs of cigarettes a day for years, quit the habit after only one session with me. He also reported no withdrawal symptoms. I will never forget my excitement as I thought, "Wow, this really works!"

My next client was Herman, a seventy-year-old man who wished to give up drinking alcohol. Sadly, his daily excessive drinking had become too much for his family to handle. His wife had divorced him decades earlier, and his children had rejected him. Not having spoken to his children in years, Herman desperately wanted a relationship with them and with his grandchildren before he died.

I told him I was quite certain I could help and conducted a hypnotherapy session with him. He easily went into a deep hypnotic trance, and I guided him to visualize and feel how great it would feel to be a nondrinker. I helped him relax further and led him to imagine and emotionally experience the hugs and happy tears of his children and grandchildren as they opened their hearts to him once again.

I gave Herman powerful hypnotic suggestions to view alcohol as the toxin it is and to feel how he would now release it easily from his life. I also led his memory back to the time in his life before he started drinking and to remember how effortless, fun, easy, and natural it was to be a nondrinker. "What once was, now is," I quietly, yet firmly, stated while he enjoyed the hypnotic state.

Herman's subconscious mind, now fully open to my suggestions and images, allowed a wonderful transformation to occur. As is true with almost all of my clients, when he opened his eyes after the session, he felt instantly refreshed, energized, and happy. At his follow-up session the next week, he came in beaming and with tearful eyes told me that from the moment he left his first session, his desire for alcohol was completely gone.

He said that all of his drinking buddies were amazed and would provide testimonials that he no longer visited the bars.

His buddy, Don, had this to say: "I've never seen Herman without a drink in his hand, and I've known him a long time. After the hypnosis, he just stopped drinking. No cravings, nothing. Pretty amazing."

Best of all, his children and grandchildren forgave him and he was now joyfully a part of their lives. Witnessing these and the other early successes, I became more and more committed to using hypnosis. It became my work focus and passion, and I began to use it in my own personal life in many wondrous ways.

■ PARTNERS IN HEALING

As a professional hypnotherapist, I consider myself a partner in my client's healing journey. Although some of my clients may need additional appointments, I continue to hold the expectation that they will be able to make significant progress within just one session.

My professional experience has led me to believe we are "all one," and therefore the relationship between the therapist and client will have different outcomes depending on the mindset of both. Therefore, one of my roles is to help each client develop an expectation of success even before I begin the hypnosis. With a mutual mindset of positive expectations, healing can, and often does, occur at an accelerated pace.

Sometimes my client's success becomes blocked by skepticism, self-blame, shame, and feelings of unworthiness. In these cases, we may decide together to address these blocks before moving forward. For instance, when a client doesn't become a complete nonsmoker in the first session, I become intrigued and know that I can find the missing link. A quick follow-up session is usually all we need to make the appropriate corrections.

As I mentioned earlier, my clients' intentions are of utmost importance to their success. I explain to them that we are entering a partnership. I cannot do anything without their approval and cooperation. In fact, I don't hypnotize anyone. They hypnotize themselves.

The techniques work, but only if the clients are willing for them to work, I explain. They must be motivated to change and be willing and able to relax. To help accomplish this, I have created a comfortable and relaxing office environment. My goal is to have people feel instant calm as soon as they enter my waiting room. I want my office to be a relaxation oasis for each and every person who enters, even for the mail carrier who drops off my daily mail!

I painted the walls a soothing blue, placed a beautiful rug on the floor, added upbeat health magazines for reading, low intensity table lighting, filtered water, and a water fountain with bird chirping sounds. First-time clients listen to my eight-minute *Introduction to Hypnosis* CD in the waiting room, which relaxes them and also serves to educate them on the "hows and whys" of hypnosis.

By the time they enter my inner office, they are usually very relaxed, ready, and prepared to have a successful session.

I invite them to relax in the soft recliner. I serve them tea or water and love to place a comfy blanket on them as they relax and let me do my work. I instruct them that I will simply guide their ever-listening subconscious mind to receive positive hypnotic suggestions, which will allow them to take control of their mind, emotions, and body. I explain that I will do all the work; all they need to do is relax and enjoy the session.

To help my clients hasten and deepen their healing, I produced a series of self-hypnosis recordings, which I now sell worldwide. I have heard from many people that simply by using my *Quit Smoking* CD, they were able to quit the habit effortlessly. For instance, I was speaking at a local health expo one year and was approached by a young woman who had purchased my *Quit Smoking* CD the earlier year. She excitedly told me that she and her college roommate listened to it every night as they fell asleep. They both quit smoking in just one week and have been nonsmokers ever since.

Another client, John, purchased my *Weight Loss Hypnosis* CD and lost six pounds in ten days. He became my client and proceeded to lose another forty pounds with individual sessions.

Hypnosis is simply using how the mind works and using the proper programming for success.

My friend, Laurel, took my *Quit Smoking* CD with her during a Hawaiian vacation. She listened to it twice daily and was a nonsmoker by day four of her vacation. That was four years ago, and she remains a nonsmoker to this day. Besides giving up smoking, my clients have discovered that they also do not gain weight. In fact, many of my clients have reported losing ten to twenty pounds as a wonderful side effect of quitting smoking with my program.

By the way, I never refer to my clients as smokers or addicts or by any other label. I see them as healthy as they were at birth, and I have yet to hear of a baby being born with a cigarette hanging from his mouth! Everyone is born a nonsmoker, as a nonaddict. They are happy, trusting, and self-loving. It's what comes after birth that programs us for addictive and self-destructive beliefs and behaviors.

With specific hypnosis techniques, I simply help people revert to their natural states of good health and healthy behaviors. I help them connect to their true essence of positive energy and vitality.

I often have prospective clients call me and say, "I know there's no quick fix." They are surprised to hear me say, "Yes there is!"

I have many years of success to back up that statement. I tell people that hypnosis can be quick, easy, pleasant, and effective. The "no quick fix" statement is just an unhelpful hypnotic or programmed statement that keeps people stuck.

My work is about getting people unstuck and moving forward with ease and happiness. After all these years, I am still amazed at how quickly the subconscious mind can be reprogrammed and how, with motivation and an open mind, we can all lead the bountiful, healthy, happy lives that we were born to enjoy.

— HOW TO USE THIS BOOK —

The book you hold in your hands can help you change your life. In fact, right this minute, go get your camera and take a picture of yourself. Then, label the photo "The Old Me." Here's my promise to you. If you do what I've outlined for you in this book, you will soon have another photo—and you will be able to proudly label it, "The Me I Was Meant to Be."

What's so different about this book, and why am I so sure it can help you when all the other things you've tried might have failed?

Here are four powerful reasons why this weight loss program will be your last:

1. The information contained in this book has been tested and proven to be successful by my clients for more than twenty years. It is also the same information I used to restore my own health and fitness after gaining more than fifty pounds and to maintain my weight loss.

2. This book focuses on *you* and your unique approach to life. It gives you not just one solution—but an entire collection of them. You will choose the methods that feel right for you, and you have the freedom to start with just one method—or combine several different options.

3. This book will guide you to make the most important changes you can make—the changes in your mind and your thoughts. How do I know this is so? My clients prove it to me every day. Many of them had only one session with me and were able to achieve and maintain their desired goal—because they were able to reprogram their minds for success.

4. This book makes it easy! I have taught these methods to teens and adults alike. Not only have my clients been successful, but they have also discovered that the journey could actually be both effective and fun.

So I wrote this book for three compelling reasons. First, I see the need for a tangible, lasting, and healthy solution to achieving weight loss. I shudder to see people spending hundreds of dollars and undergoing needless emotional trauma while failing at weight loss programs.

According to the World Health Organization, over 1.5 billion adults are overweight and of these, over 500 million are obese. And although millions of dollars are spent daily on weight loss, sadly, people across the globe are getting heavier and unhealthier.

The second reason I wrote this book is that the majority of weight loss "solutions" do not offer effective road maps. The typical road map includes external changes, supplements (some of them dangerous), or radical behavior modification that, by its very nature, cannot be sustained.

The road map that will get you where you want to go begins in your mind. Your thoughts determine the direction and the rules of the road.

Even better news? Once you understand how to reprogram your mind for weight loss success, you can program your mind in the same manner for all other changes you may want to make: reducing stress, quitting smoking, enjoying more confidence, improving your finances, even finding your mate!

It all begins in your mind, and this book can be as powerful a tool as you wish to make it.

And that's the third reason I wrote this book. I want you to experience lasting success with your weight loss journey and build happy memories as you do so.

> *When you change the way you look at things,*
> *the things you look at change.* — DR. WAYNE DYER

It is said that you only need to change 3 percent of what you are doing, for the rest of your life to begin changing. Use this book to change how you see your weight loss journey. View this journey as an exciting adventure of personal growth. See yourself walking your new path with joy and anticipation. And keep that camera nearby. The New You is very close!

■ HOW TO USE THIS BOOK TO CHANGE YOUR LIFE

As a counselor, I have found that the most lasting and profound changes can be made when they are easy, fun, and experiential. This book is designed with this in mind; for you to experience the *joy* and *ease* of reaching your weight goals and maintaining your success.

There are various ways to use this book:

1. Privately: Immerse yourself in a powerful, loving, intimate workshop of self-discovery and healing as you become the slender and healthy person you were meant to be. This book is your personal workbook. Start at the beginning and go chapter by chapter. Or, let your intuition guide you on which chapters to focus on. Some chapters may call for you to linger a while, really mastering the theme. Take your time. Remember, this is the last time you will need to lose weight, as your weight loss will be permanent!

2. With friends, family, or colleagues: This book can serve as a wonderful book club focus or as a weight loss support group guide. The power of group consciousness with the combined intention of health and happiness cannot be overemphasized.

Whether you choose to take this exciting journey alone or with others is entirely your choice. There is no right or wrong way. The important thing is to start.

Part I of this book focuses on the emotional nature of eating and how to let go of emotional addiction to food. This will include:

• Simple self-awareness exercises
• Affirmations for success
• Self-esteem building tools
• Transformational manifestation steps
• Powerful visualizations
• Guided imagery scripts
• Effective hypnosis techniques
• Motivational stories that you can make your own
• Success journal entries for structure and note taking

All of these will help you attain emotional freedom from food and make your journey a pleasant and easy one. I simply do not subscribe to the myth that positive changes need to be difficult and time consuming. One of the many reasons I've embraced guided imagery and hypnotherapy is that changes can be accomplished quickly and in an easy and pleasant manner. Once you've released emotional and behavioral barriers, such as feelings of unworthiness, negative self-talk, and other damaging and limiting attitudes, you're free to become the person of your dreams.

I encourage you to use my *Hypnosis for Weight Loss* CD, which is a wonderful complement to this book. Using these techniques in the book, along with the power of hypnosis in the CD, you can begin to make changes right away.

You can get results similar to Lauren from Cedar Rapids, Iowa, who wrote:

Your weight loss CD is just amazing. I can't believe what has happened. I realized I never really tasted food before. Now I savor and chew every bite and I need to eat less. Food even smells wonderful, which I never used to notice. I can see a bag of potato chips, and it means nothing to me! At our holiday baking day with friends, I enjoyed the baking but had no desire to eat any of the cookies. Now, instead of eating chocolate and cookies every afternoon, I relax with your CD. I feel so energized without all that sugar!

Part II of this book will provide you with essential facts about food, eating habits, and exercise, and their effects on metabolism, cravings, and weight gain. You don't need to know every nook and cranny of nutrition, but I do believe that without this basic knowledge you may not be as successful as you'd like to be on your weight loss journey. I am not a nutritionist, doctor, or dietician, so I have not gone into a scholarly analysis of the nutritional aspects and chemical nature of food. I have, however, done a lot of research into nutrition and will share with you the basics of the research I've read and the success stories of people I know (including myself) who have learned which foods and additives to avoid for health reasons.

For those of you who would like more information, I have provided excellent resources on healthy food in the appendix.

Although the main focus of this book is on weight loss, it is also intended to help you see how you can, by shifting your mental focus and intention, alter every aspect of your life: become a nonsmoker, gain the confidence to get a great job, develop your athletic skills, tap into your creative genius, and learn to relax. There is no limit to the things that can be accomplished with focus and attention.

To help you see the fabulous benefits and potentials available, I will provide you with stories and testimonials of my clients who have used my techniques to gain the self-control, motivation, and ability to live the life of their dreams. I have also written of my own weight loss journey. In fact, this book began years ago in the form of my personal diary entries. The results I got were so significant that I eventually felt compelled to share my discoveries with everyone.

Remember this: There is no rush.

As a note of encouragement to you, Dear Reader, I'd like you to remember to always treat yourself with kindness during your weight loss journey. When you keep in mind that you are losing weight for life, you will realize that you have time. There is no need to push yourself or to hurry the process. In fact, when you view this process as the last time you lose weight, you can allow yourself time to enjoy the journey. Savor the process. Say good-bye forever to each pound you lose, and say hello to being thin forever!

Imagine this: One of my favorite hypnotic images to help clients lose weight is to suggest that they are a part of nature, like a beautiful plant growing in a green meadow. I guide them to imagine the slender stalks of wheat, thin blades of grass, and graceful, lean stems of flowers. Plants are surrounded by nourishment in the soil, but only take the exact amount necessary for beauty, strength, and health. "You are like the slender, perfect flower stem. You take in the proper nourishment and leave the rest," I suggest. "There is no need to overconsume or to hoard food. You are slender, strong, trim, and perfect."

I encourage you to adopt this image of a beautiful plant as inspiration to achieve and enjoy the healthy body of your dreams ... the healthy, slender body that you deserve.

PART I

Letting Go of Emotional Eating

CHAPTER 1

Awareness is the greatest agent for change.

—ECKHART TOLLE

How I Found
the Weight Loss Solution

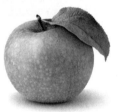

FOR YEARS,

I WENT ABOUT

LOSING WEIGHT in ways that caused me to lose the weight, only to gain it back again, known as the yo-yo syndrome. I often felt cravings and deprivation. I would be miserable until I lost some weight and then started eating all the wrong foods again, only to gain the weight back in record time. The good news is that I found the solutions, and this book is about sharing them with you. This book is also about helping you with a sound, emotionally positive plan to lose your weight and keep it off, while successfully avoiding feelings of deprivation and cravings.

In my 25 years as a counselor, I've observed two main reasons why people have a hard time reaching their weight goals:

- *One,* they don't have the correct information about food, cravings, and metabolism.
- *Two,* they are emotionally dependent upon food.

I've discovered that for weight loss to be successful and permanent, both issues must be addressed. When I simply helped people sever their dysfunctional emotional ties with food, their physical bodies still craved unhealthy food because of toxicity, inflammation, and the addiction to harmful chemicals found in many food products today. I have found that nutritionally detoxifying the body, especially the liver, is as important to weight loss as is letting go of the emotional addiction. This is very similar to the process when we seek emotional healing. First, we must "detoxify" faulty belief systems, and then we can implant newer, healthier ones.

It took me several years of weight fluctuations and considerable frustration before I discovered the healthy way to permanently lose weight.

I want to help you avoid the same frustration. It is my desire to help you reach your weight loss goals in a much shorter and simpler way than I did. Part of my problem was that we simply didn't have the information years ago that we have now about metabolism and chemical addiction to foods. Today, holistic doctors of functional medicine are making this information widely accessible and understandable. Because of this new branch of medicine, I have been able to research and use sound medical advice to help me heal from metabolic disorders.

Paired with my expertise in releasing emotional addiction to food, I have been able to adhere to a plan that has allowed me to reach a weight I never thought would be possible in my fifties. It is never too late to become healthy, fit, and slender. I'm living proof of that.

Traditional diets deal primarily with calorie restriction. By eating fewer calories than you burn, you will lose weight. However, this process is often very difficult to stick with and sustain. Why? Because the emotional component is missing—and without addressing the emotional issues relating to food, most people have a very difficult time feeling happy and strong while dieting.

With traditional dieting, people engage their conscious willpower to forcefully eat less until they lose the weight. Then, success in hand, they often go back to the unhealthy eating habits that caused them to gain weight in the first place.

Look at the celebrities who have publicly aired their weight loss struggles of losing and gaining weight. They have all the resources in the world to help them stay fit, including personal trainers, fabulous budgets for private gyms, and all the latest written studies on how to lose weight. But, clearly, they too have hidden issues that keep them from maintaining their weight loss once they achieve it.

This is because willpower, although strong at times, is severely limited in how long it can sustain difficult behavior changes. This is especially true when it comes to food, which is plentiful and pleasantly displayed in stores and constantly in our faces with TV commercials, billboards, and print advertising.

It makes my heart sad to see candy and other sugary treats displayed throughout the grocery stores in most every aisle. Even if you've managed to ignore it until checkout time, the candy temptation appears yet again as you place your food purchases on the conveyor belt.

It takes an extreme amount of willpower to not cave in to these sugar triggers. Unfortunately, many of us succumb and begin a downward spiral from Halloween through New Year's Day. Many people make a New Year's resolution to get off the sugar and overeating habit and do well during the month of January. This only lasts a couple of weeks until the Valentine's Day commercials for chocolate begin to bombard us! If you're emotionally or physically addicted to sugar, you'll have a very hard time ignoring the candy advertisements and will feel like a failure as you continue to surrender to your cravings.

▪ THE STATE FAIR SYNDROME

I've lived in Minnesota for thirty years and have spent the majority of those years living within walking distance of our remarkable state fairgrounds. The state fair runs for twelve days, ending on Labor Day. Throughout the summer months, TV and billboard advertising promote the "Great Minnesota Get Together," enticing us with photographs of delectable food, most of which is dipped in grease or sugar and served conveniently on a stick. If you've ever been to a state or county fair, you know that it's one big fast food haven. Greasy, sugary, fatty foods are everywhere and the aroma is so enticing. In fact, one of the commercials advertising the fair states that "It's all about the food!"

Although there are many wonderful aspects to the fair, such as watching baby animals being born and visiting the home improvement, agriculture, crafts, education, and technology booths, the big draw is the food. I even have clients see me for hypnosis sessions in August for help in controlling their cravings during their state fair visit.

Why is this a syndrome? Well, I've observed that when people gather for a social event they tend to feel it's totally acceptable to overeat together. We see this dramatically played out on Thanksgiving Day, for example. When we're all doing it together, it almost feels as though it won't hurt us. It's as though these special calories consumed during holidays, festivals, and celebration, magically don't count! People go into the illusion of addictive eating together and later suffer the unhappy consequences of weight gain alone.

As a counselor, I help people let go of such illusions and embrace truth. By living in truth we can find self-control and achieve and maintain our goals.

Changing your eating behaviors is not about an extreme diet to temporarily lose weight for that cruise or for an upcoming wedding. It's time to stop the yo-yo pattern and get healthy and fit for life. It is my fervent wish and genuine intention to help you attain your weight and health goals in a pleasant, easy, and permanent way.

In my workshops and individual sessions, I invite people to learn how to crack the code to weight issues. By addressing both the physical and emotional components inherent in a weight problem, my clients become truly liberated from food addiction and permanently enjoy the body shape, size, and weight of their dreams.

> *This is a success that you as the reader can certainly attain for yourself as well.*

CHAPTER 2

If I desire change I must first look to my own mind.

—LEE JAMPOLSKY

My Story... Your Story

Weight Gain Begins in the Mind

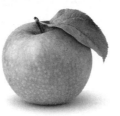

MUCH TO

THE AMAZEMENT

OF EVERYONE, MY MOTHER gave birth to four consecutive and healthy sets of twins, and one single child, all within eight years! My twin brother, Ken, and I were the second set of twins. Being so close in age, the nine of us were constant companions, enjoying all forms of sports together. I loved growing up in upstate New York, ice skating and sledding in the winter and swimming during the hot summer months. I was effortlessly thin as a child, as were my eight brothers and sisters.

Although food was abundant in our house-

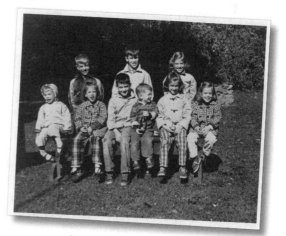

Can you pair each set of twins?
(The author is seated second from the right)

hold, it was never the center of attention. Everyday meals for our family of eleven were cooked by Mom, with the special Sunday and holiday meals prepared by Dad. Similar to other housewives in the 1950s, Mom's dinner preparation depended on a daily schedule. Although I don't remember what the schedule was for all of the days of the week, I do remember Hungarian Goulash on Mondays and fish sticks on Fridays.

On Sunday, Mom took the nine children to church while Dad stayed behind to cook a special meal. We also took turns having Sunday meals at Grandma and Grandpa's house. Our family was so blessed to have two grandmas who were both outstanding cooks. Our paternal grandma, a Slovenian immigrant, was a superb cook who always served delicious, savory meals with lots of vegetables. Her specialties were chicken noodle soup with homemade noodles and strudel.

Our maternal grandma, whom we called Babci, was an excellent Polish cook who spoiled us with delectable cabbage rolls, home-canned fruit, fresh vegetables, and pastries. Some of my happiest childhood moments were celebrating religious holidays at our grandparents' homes, enjoying the elaborate feasts that took weeks to prepare. These meals, including sugary treats, were greatly anticipated special events.

Everyday fare was unspectacular, although healthy. Eating was for basic nutrition, not a source of entertainment or relief from boredom. After all, with eight brothers and sisters, life was seldom boring!

In looking back on my childhood, I discovered that we tended to stay naturally thin for four reasons:

1. We were constantly active in sports and creative activities. We walked or biked everywhere. TV was a very minor part of the day. And, of course, household computers and video games were not even conceived of yet.

2. Meals were eaten at the kitchen or dining room tables, never in front of the television. It was fun sitting down together every day when Dad came home from work.

3. Desserts were reserved for special celebrations. They were not everyday indulgences. We snacked on the fruit that was in constant supply. This is in contrast to current lifestyle habits of eating sweets and huge meals on a daily basis.

4. We rarely ate at restaurants. There was the occasional fish fry on Friday nights during Lent or a very occasional McDonald's stop. (We each got one hamburger and one small fry. Thankfully, this was before the days of Super Size Me!)

■ COLLEGE YEARS

I stayed thin throughout my childhood and college years. Obesity was simply not an issue for most of us. My college roommates were very thin, and I remember lots of fun discussions at the dormitory dining hall. One day, our lively discussion turned to the topic of quirky eating habits. I was amazed to hear my good friend, Natalie, say, "I have this thing that I have to eat everything off my plate. I can't leave food, even if I'm full."

This was such a strange concept to me! To my horror, I felt her words seeping into my mind, like water soaking parched earth, as I instantly wondered, "What if this happened to me?" This was my personal introduction to the power of hypnotic suggestion. Because I admired Natalie and loved her as a dear friend, I was at a heightened state of suggestion when she shared her food struggle, and as she did so, her food issue instantly became my issue. As hard as I fought them off, her words haunted me and made meal times much harder. Before that moment, I never even thought of overeating as a possibility. After all, we were never admonished for not eating all our food at home. We ate until we felt satisfied and then were excused from the table.

I was able to stay thin throughout graduate school, but the pull of overeating was annoyingly consistent. Sharing food was becoming more and more a social pastime, and I had to consciously hold back from overeating. Fortunately, I had fallen in love with taking ballet classes. The mindfulness of this form of athletic movement to beautiful music was extremely therapeutic for me. Entering the ballet studio was like walking into a stunning fantasy world. It was quiet, peaceful, and elegant. I felt proud of my thin body and was motivated to stay svelte as a ballet student. The mirror-lined studio made it impossible to not be aware of my body shape and size. Ballet is quite strenuous, so there was no crash dieting for me. I just ate healthy foods in appropriate quantities.

As a professional woman after graduate school, I kept my weight at a healthy level by keeping up the ballet classes. I also had very little money, so eating at restaurants remained a foreign concept to me. My first place of employment was as a counselor at a sheltered workshop for handicapped adults. It was a beautiful modern facility with a large kitchen and cooking staff, and I enjoyed healthy meals with my colleagues and clients. Before and after work, I relaxed by walking my Irish Setter/Black Lab dog, Molly. Dinner was cheap and simple: often a can of soup heated up. On weekends, Molly and I would take wonderful, long walks around the many Minnesota lakes or along the Mississippi River. These walks with Molly, and my ballet classes were my therapy. My weight stayed under 120 pounds effortlessly.

■ *MISCARRIAGES AND WEIGHT GAIN*

I fell in love and was married at age 26. It was exciting to think about forming a new family, and my husband and I anticipated pregnancy with joyful expectation. Sadly, we were faced with a series of heartbreaking miscarriages and the prospect of not bearing children together. Although we were elated for our friends and relatives who were having babies, it was agonizing to get birth announcements from them. I felt determined to do anything to have a successful pregnancy and decided to put on a few pounds just in case my thinness was one of the problems.

Finally conceiving again after two miscarriages, I began reading as many books about nutrition in pregnancy as I could get my hands on. Desperately wanting a full-term pregnancy, I gave myself permission to eat copious amounts of food to ensure proper nutrition for my unborn child. To my elation, I gave birth to my wonderful son Bernard, and 21 months later, to his adorable brother, Joseph. Although I was able to lose the pregnancy weight after both births, a few years later I started to suddenly and rapidly gain weight. My weight ballooned up fifty pounds, and to my horror I was at my full-term pregnancy weight without being pregnant!

I heard this same sad story from so many of my female weight loss clients that I started to question why returning exactly to the pregnancy weight, years after the last pregnancy ended, was so commonplace. The prevailing theory at the time suggested that a woman's highest adult weight, no matter how short-lived, can become an established new biological set weight that is difficult, if not impossible, to reset. This was terrifying and unacceptable to me.

Seeing how so many women tended to return to and stay stuck at their highest pregnancy weight, years after the pregnancies ended, seemed too coincidental to overlook. I wondered if the subconscious mind had a role in this mysterious occurrence. Delving into this during counseling sessions with my female clients, I discovered that many of these women, like me, had suffered miscarriages and considered their successful pregnancies to be the times of their most extreme joy.

For many of these women, their happiest memories were of being in the last trimester of pregnancy. I became convinced that during pregnancy, whether or not miscarriages were involved, the subconscious mind had equated the act of eating large amounts of food with the emotion of happiness. Could the subconscious mind have equated overeating and gaining weight with life, survival and happiness? If so, then, in the future, whenever we felt sad, hopeless, or felt any other feelings of despair, the subconscious mind's programming prompted us to unconsciously eat large quantities of food as a means of feeling better. It made us feel in control.

I even remember feeling strangely safe and happy when my abdomen was large, similar to how I looked at five months pregnant! Even though I wanted to be thin again, I seemed hopelessly blocked. Whenever I tried to diet, a huge inner wall stopped my efforts and I would soon sabotage and abandon my weight loss plan.

With this insight and a strong desire to lose weight, I hypnotized myself to permanently sever the connection of overeating from feelings of happiness and control.

■ *MY SELF-HYPNOSIS SUCCESS*

I reprogrammed my subconscious mind with this thought: *Although the happy months of pregnancy are over, I will continue to experience tremendous joy as a mother... as a healthy, slim mother!* By giving myself the powerful hypnotic suggestion that the joy of pregnancy and giving birth was totally unrelated to overeating and gaining weight, I was on my way to freeing myself from the subconscious drive to eat from emotional need.

I paired this suggestion with visualizing myself happily enjoying my children, with a flat abdomen and slender body. This was a major, and necessary, step forward on my weight loss journey and has served as a vital part of my skills as a weight loss counselor.

With this awakening, I immediately began helping women permanently sever the unconscious connection of food and pregnancy happiness. And it worked!

I began applying these discoveries to everyone who came to see me about their particular problems and was pleased to find that these insights were successful in almost all circumstances, no matter what life event had been associated with emotional eating.

■ *Jim's Story: Former Athelete*

Like many men, Jim enjoyed exhilarating years as a high school athlete. In fact, he still enjoys hanging out after work with his high school buddies, drinking beer, and reminiscing about the good old days as football heroes.

"I used to be able to eat as much as I wanted back then," he said. "Football was my life, and I had to eat lots of burgers and fries to stay bulked up and powerful." Things changed for Jim, however, when he became a husband and father. "My eating seems out of control, and I now have a big gut instead of great abs." The problem, I told Jim, was not due to a lack of willpower, but to faulty programming in the memory archives of his mind. Using hypnosis, I was able to help Jim stop unconsciously associating overeating with the thrill of bygone days and reclaim a strong motivation and ability to become a fit thirty-four-year-old man.

I began to think, "If happy events have the power to keep us stuck in the habit of overeating, what power do painful events have?"

■ *PAINFUL MEMORIES AND WEIGHT GAIN*

This led me to look at how painful life events could produce faulty subconscious programming and trigger weight gain years after a major life event had occurred.

Whenever a weight loss client told me that he or she had been thin during youth but then gained weight that stubbornly wouldn't come off, I began asking *"What was going on in your life right before the weight gain started?"*

■ *Danielle*

Upon hearing this question, my weight loss client, Danielle, got an instant vision of jogging along the Mississippi River walking path. With a smile, she said, "I loved running every day. I was thin and athletic. I've tried so hard to get back into running, but I feel like something is blocking me."

I then asked, "Did anything traumatic happen to you around this time of life?" Danielle's eyes filled with tears as she remembered that her brother, with whom she was very close, had been tragically killed in a car accident. She felt heartbroken for a long time after his death. I told her that I now had the information I needed to help her and shared the insight that her subconscious mind had wrongly associated her brother's death with her healthy lifestyle.

Her subconscious mind, I explained, was trying to protect her from further trauma by keeping her overweight. Danielle responded with, "That's crazy!" Many of my clients have that same reaction. I explained that the subconscious mind is not logical, but operates only with images and emotions. It automatically pairs and remembers events with strings of emotional states no matter how irrational and illogical these connections may be.

As strange as it sounds, Danielle's subconscious mind was operating as though her brother's death was related to her superb fitness level!

With Danielle's permission, I relaxed her into a state of hypnosis and gave her subconscious mind the suggestion that her brother's death had absolutely no connection to her being thin and athletic.

I then took her to happy memories during her life while she was enjoying jogging as a lean, healthy woman. Thus, I grounded an association of exercise and healthy eating with the feeling states of happiness, self-control, safety, and pride.

A few weeks after her session, Danielle reported that not only did she feel remarkably "free and happy," but also that she found herself eating less and had actually started running again. She said she had a new goal of running a marathon and was confident that she would reach that goal.

■ Robert

I remember another client, Robert, who, like Danielle, struggled with a lack of motivation to lose weight. At a younger, thinner time of life, he often enjoyed relaxing after work by biking through a favorite city park. Things changed abruptly one evening, however, when a man jumped out from the bushes, violently pushed Robert off his bike, beat him, and stole his wallet. Although he felt he had long ago emotionally healed from this traumatic event, his subconscious mind was still unconsciously operating under the mistaken and irrational view that the attack was associated with being thin. With this insight, Robert was able to release this association during a light hypnotic state. I paired feelings of safety and calm with images of his healthy, slender body. Like so many of my clients, Robert was now free to lose the weight that had mysteriously plagued him for so many years.

■ Angela

Just the other day, a new client named Angela entered my office for a weight loss session. She told me how she had been "effortlessly thin" all of her life, barely ever reaching 115 pounds, until her late thirties. At age 46 and just under 5 feet tall, her 180 current pounds was causing her a multitude of painful ailments, including Type 2 diabetes and arthritis.

Although her doctor and girlfriends told her it was probably aging hormones that kept her stuck, Angela suspected something else was to blame. I agreed with her suspicion and asked if some traumatic life event occurred right before she started gaining weight. This question prompted Angela to sob.

Reaching for the tissue box, Angela tearfully recounted how her husband had an affair when she was thirty-six-years old, breaking her heart and ending their marriage. Even though this event had occurred several years ago, the memory of it still caused her terrible grief and anger. I explained to Angela that she, like most of us, innocently turned to food for emotional comfort during that difficult time. More importantly, I said, her subconscious mind had wrongly and irrationally associated being thin with her husband's infidelity. As long as she stayed overweight, I suggested, the illusion her subconscious mind created allowed her to feel safe from being cheated on again. Happily, after just a few sessions, Angela was able to restore a subconscious association of safety and inner strength with being thin and was well on her way to shedding the excess pounds.

Although there is never just one explanation for complex emotional issues, I have found that faulty subconscious programming due to past life events, both happy and painful, is often a cause for stubborn weight gain issues. By addressing the programming, which always occurs innocently enough, we can free ourselves from the physical bondage of extra pounds and inches. This is not to say, however, that all weight gain arises from significant life events. Sometimes weight slowly creeps up as our lives become more sedentary, such as when we work in an office environment. Stay-at-home parents and people who work from a home office often gain weight simply because the kitchen is in close proximity and unhealthy snacking becomes a daily habit. It takes just an extra fifty calories a day, which is the equivalent of a half piece of bread or one small cookie, to gain ten pounds a year.

* **A Note About the Success Journal Entries:** *Journaling is a time-honored means of exploring an idea and reinforcing a resolution. The physical act of writing etches an idea deep in your experiential memories. However, this is your personal weight loss experience. If you prefer to not write now (or at all), take a moment to simply mentally ponder the questions. Or, if the reading of the text is flowing and you wish to continue, feel free to come back to the journal at another time.*

SUCCESS JOURNAL ENTRY: *Your Story*

At what point in your life did you begin to gain weight?

_____

_____

_____

*Was there a significant life event, positive or negative,
that occurred right before your weight gain began?*

_____

_____

_____

_____

*Remind yourself that your body shape, weight, and size, along with your
eating habits, were unrelated to the event itself. Imagine dealing with
that life event differently. Write down how that would look.*

_____

_____

_____

_____

_____

Visualize yourself slender, fit, and healthy starting today.

CHAPTER 3

Decisions are doorways to change.
—TONY ROBBINS

Making the Decision to Change

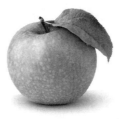

THE FIRST STEP

TO LOSING WEIGHT

AND GETTING HEALTHY is the most important step. It is to decide. Stop the denial. Stop the excuses. *Decide* to have the body you want today. Without firm commitment, life stress, excuses, and inner sabotage will flood in and block permanent weight loss. I want to help you feel motivated and make a strong commitment to changing your eating habits. Are you ready to decide and commit to having the body you deserve and desire? Are you ready to stop the yo-yo frustration?

Like most people who need to lose weight, I used to think "I'll be happier once I lose weight." Try changing this to: *"As I get happier, I'll lose weight."*

Your primary goal is happiness and maintaining good, vibrant health. What makes you happy? Is it being overweight, sick, and tired or being healthy with lots of energy to enjoy fun activities? As extra pounds creep in, the human body becomes more and more sluggish. The more sluggish you become, the activities that once gave you so much joy diminish one by one. Life can begin to feel very constrained.

■ *POWERING UP YOUR MOTIVATION TO CHANGE*

As a weight loss coach, I find it essential to help my clients tap into, grow, and stay connected with their motivation to lose weight. Without continuous motivation, any weight loss plan can fizzle out pretty quickly. I find it helpful to explore with them how being overweight limits them and how losing weight will enhance their lives.

In response to my question, *"What brings you in today?"* I hear things like this:

- *I can't play with my toddler and preschooler. I just can't keep up.*

- *I'm tired of being the most overweight one in my group of friends.*

- *I feel so out of control. Food and a huge appetite control me.*

- *My clothes are so uncomfortable and tight. Elastic waistbands embarrass me.*

- *I feel tired all of the time, no matter how much sleep I get.*

- *I'm on blood pressure medication, and I'm only 30 years old!*

- *My doctor says I'm prediabetic. This scares me!*

- *I'm afraid of dying before my kids grow up.*

- *I feel unattractive and old looking. The double chin and potbelly really bother me.*

- *I hate summer because I can't wear shorts and sleeveless dresses.*

- *I'm frustrated and angry with myself for gaining so much weight.*

- *I sleep and watch TV too much. The extra pounds make me feel lazy.*

- *I hate the brain fog! My memory and focus are shot!*

- *I'm addicted to sugar. I can't imagine not eating it every day.*

- *I barely squeeze into restaurant booths and airplane seats. It's so uncomfortable.*

- *I can't bend down to tie my shoes.*

- *I feel ashamed of myself for letting my weight get this out of control.*

I tell my clients: *"Turn the negatives into positive goals. It's best to focus on what you want, rather than on what you dislike."* For example:

• *I want to keep up with my kids when they're running around the playground.*

• *I want to fit in with my thin friends.*

• *I want to be in control of what, when, and how much I eat.*

• *I want my clothes to fit loosely and to be able to button the waist button.*

• *I want to feel energetic, youthful, and happy.*

• *I want to cut down on or eliminate my medications.*

• *I want to be healthy.*

• *I want to live a long, fulfilling life and see my children grow up.*

• *I want to look in the mirror and feel proud of how I look.*

• *I want to look attractive wearing summer clothes.*

• *I want to feel satisfied with how I look and feel.*

• *I want to be active again, like I was in my twenties.*

• *I want a clear and focused mind.*

• *I want to have a "take it or leave it" attitude toward sweets.*

• *I want to feel comfortable sitting at restaurant booths and on planes and movie theater seats.*

• *I want to bend down easily to tie my shoes.*

• *I want to get my self-esteem back and lose the shame.*

The next step is to *know* that reaching your weight loss goals will allow you to do these things. Now, *imagine* how great it will feel to be living the healthy, fit life you were born to enjoy!

When you focus on being happy and enjoying life, such as seeing friends, going to movies, dancing, and enjoying hobbies, you'll have a more complete picture of what losing weight means to you. *It's not about the number on the scale and dieting, but about living a fulfilling and fun life.*

SUCCESS JOURNAL ENTRY

*Use this worksheet to help you identify your thoughts about your weight
and ways to begin changing those thoughts into supportive ones.
Keeping a weight journal about your changing thoughts and your progress
is another fabulous way to support yourself as you choose to change
and become the best you that you can be.*

HOW BEING OVERWEIGHT LIMITS ME:

PHYSICALLY.
*Example: "I feel sluggish and exhausted all day.
All I can do is sit and watch TV."*

_____

_____

MENTALLY.
Example: "My memory is shot. I can't think straight."

_____

_____

EMOTIONALLY.
Example: "I hate looking in the mirror. It makes me feel like a failure."

_____

_____

CHANGE EACH LIMITATION INTO DESIRE AFFIRMATIONS.
Example: "I want to feel energized all day."

_____

_____

_____

_____

Now, visualize yourself achieving your goals with ease and confidence. Keep negative statements and doubt away!

Feel proud for making the decision to get healthy. Be proud of being a picky grocery shopper, a picky eater, of caring for your body. Without a healthy body, you cannot live an active life.

Tell yourself: *"Reaching these goals is in my best interest and in the best interest of everyone I come into contact with. I deserve to reach my health goals. I enjoy getting fit and healthy, today and from this day forward."*

Your goal is to change your mindset. First, identify what you do want, record it in your journal, and use visualization to imagine you are already there.

Look within! ...The secret is inside you.

—HUI-NENG

Connect with the Thin, Fabulous You

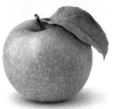

ONE THING

I'VE LEARNED

OVER THE MANY YEARS as a weight loss counselor is that it's next to impossible to lose weight and permanently keep it off if you continue to identify with an overweight image of yourself. Why? It's simply because you think, act, and feel as the person you subconsciously believe that you are. Even if you've lost weight with a traditional diet or gastric bypass surgery, you could very well gain the weight back if you don't firmly and permanently align your identity with that of a thin person.

> *Once your inner self and outer self agree about the truth of who you are (thin and healthy), you are in congruence and able to achieve and maintain weight loss.*

One of the most important steps to getting and staying thin is to permanently connect with your Inner Thin Person. This is not an image of a movie star or runway model. It is an image of the Real You, you as a thin person. If you've identified yourself as an overweight person, it is necessary to shift your focus. Go on a treasure hunt, and find the Thin You. She or he exists right now and is waiting to be discovered by you.

Many of my clients have a hard time finding the thin person inside because they've been labeled as fat, heavy or obese, for far too long. Sadly, they may have also been labeled as lazy or unmotivated. Labels disable, meaning that negative labels can keep us locked in a box of false identity. If you've been burdened with any of these negative labels, especially as a child, you might have absorbed and accepted them as your truth. It's time to let go of the labels that define you as anything other than healthy, motivated, slender, and fit! Remember that, regardless of your current weight issues, you do have a Thin You inside, waiting to be acknowledged.

■ POSITIVE LABELS STRENGTHEN YOU

How do you start this important step toward remembering the Thin You? If you can, get a photo of yourself when you were at a healthy weight. If you need to go all the way back to a photo of you as a child, that is fine. Any photo of you as a thin person will do. Keep it with you and look at it often. Put it on your refrigerator, your bathroom mirror, near your computer monitor, on the dashboard of your car.

Tell yourself: *"This is the real me."* If you don't have an actual photo of yourself to use you can create one in your mind. Even if you were overweight as a child, I want you to have a different image of yourself from now on. Remember, what your mind sees and believes is more important than anything else.

■ CREATING A MENTAL PHOTO

- Close your eyes and conjure up an imaginary image of yourself as a thin person. Connect with this image.

- See yourself wearing small size clothing, having a flat stomach and slender arms and legs.

- Get acquainted with this new image. (If this is difficult for you, don't despair. With practice and motivation you will be able to connect with a healthier you.)

- If your mind is not yet ready to imagine yourself within an image of thinness, think of the healthy weight you'd like to be. Place that number inside your body, perhaps in the abdominal region of your body. Imagine an outline of what a person at that weight looks like and watch that outline form around the number. Give that outline your flesh, face, and name. Now feel this thin person residing within you. Take a mental photo of her or him and use this as your vision of your Inner You, your Inner Visionary, from now on.

I used both the photos of the thin me and the meditation technique I'm about to describe to lose my weight and to keep it off. I still look at my thin photos from the past. I use them in my present life as a reminder of who I really am, and the ability of my body to stay healthy and slender.

■ MEDITATION TO CONNECT WITH THE THIN YOU

The purpose of the following meditation is to connect you to the thin, healthy person inside and to have a conversation with that person. When I first did the meditation, I was very surprised with the information I received. Old, repressed memories of how I lived and stayed thin began to surface. I was amazed at how the years I dedicated to raising children slowly began to hide my former thin self from my awareness. I had lost touch with the healthy person I used to be and with her lifestyle habits. By once again connecting with my former thin self, however, I began to remember her habits, her way of living. For instance, I remembered that when I was thin, I used to be very attentive to what I ate. I ate most of my calories early in the day rather than in the later part of the day, I exercised a bit every day, and I never had a weight problem. Food was a necessity, not a highlight, of my day.

I had very little money to spend on fast food or restaurants, so I prepared most of my meals at home. My portions were small since I was only cooking for myself. When I connected with this memory, it was like connecting with a long-lost friend. I wanted to be that thin, healthy person again and saw that it was entirely attainable.

If I lived a healthy life once, I certainly could do it again.

I asked myself, *"How can I incorporate my Inner Thin Person's advice into my life today?"* I remembered that ballet class was fun for me because it was a social time, as well as an exercise time.

So I joined Curves for Women and began to tone my body. It was difficult at first, but it got easier as I gained strength and stamina. The Thin Person inside of me was yearning for movement, and it was her voice that I now listened to.

As my fat began to melt away, the voice that told me "Eat!" also began to vanish.

I bought a full-length mirror and looked at myself honestly, unclothed or in underwear. I practiced unconditional self-love at every glance and renewed a commitment to continue to lose the fat I was seeing in the mirror. The mirror, along with my scale, became my indispensable partners in success. The mirror and scale don't lie, and I needed to see the truth in order to reach my goal.

I needed to see the truth in order to reach my goal: The mirror and my scale became my indispensable partners in success.

I had had enough of illusions, phony excuses, and lies—all coming from myself. I imagined myself as a skilled sculptor, lovingly chiseling away the outer layers of marble to reveal an attractive, slender figure. The true me, the Thin Me, was slowly emerging.

These techniques were so powerful for me and for my clients that I have used them in my workshops. I'm sure it will be just as wonderful for you to connect with your Inner Thin Person waiting to be acknowledged, heard, and revealed. Like me, you might be connecting with a thin adult image of yourself, or you may have to connect with an image of yourself as a child.

If you've had lifelong weight issues, connect with an imaginary thin person. The important thing is to get an image or a feeling of an inner vision of good health. *Even people who have had a weight problem since childhood or have never been thin still have a thin person inside.*

— *The Meditation*—

You can practice the following steps just as I've given them here, or change them to fit your needs and to better serve you. It's your tool to use as you wish, as often as you wish. Make it uniquely your own.

1. Get a photo of yourself when you were at an ideal body weight. (If you don't have a photo, skip to the next step). Look at the photo and say to yourself or out loud, *"This is the real me."* After looking at the photo for a while, go to step 3.

2. If you don't own a photo of yourself as a thin person, close your eyes and connect with the Inner Thin You. This is the slender, healthy, fit, lean person hidden within. Use the techniques outlined earlier; imagine an image of this person in your mind's eye, and hold that vision.

3. Now that you have a mind's eye photo and vision of the Thin You, close your eyes and gently focus on that vision. Recognize that this person is not devoid of issues or stress, but that he/she deals with life's challenges without food. Food for this person is not for stress relief, reward, boredom relief, medication, or mindless activity. This person eats healthily to enjoy an energized life.

4. Ask this Thin You: *"How do you stay thin? What do you eat? How much do you eat? When do you eat? How active are you? How would you advise others to become thin and healthy?"* Open your mind and heart to hear the answers. Sit or lie in silence while you receive the answers. Do not block what you are receiving with excuses and other thoughts such as, *"That won't work for me," "I'm too old now to lose weight," "That's too hard,"* or *"I can't do that."* Stay open and non-defensive. When you're ready, ask, *"What else can you tell me that will help and allow me to permanently lose weight?"* Then just listen and do not censor.

5. Imagine taking notes from this communication and living the advice you were given. Watch yourself following this advice with commitment, pride, and determination, as though you're seeing yourself on a movie screen. See yourself happy as you shed the pounds and gain energy, confidence, strength, and health. Perhaps see yourself reducing or eliminating prescription drugs, running a marathon, or shopping for smaller sized clothes, as your body has attained good health and vitality. Feel how proud you feel to be in control of what, when, and how you eat.

6. Keep daily lines of communication open with your Thin You. When you feel tempted to overeat, to eat junk food, or to lie on the couch instead of exercising, ask your Inner Visionary to guide you and prompt you to stay on track. Perhaps the voice will sound very strong and rather demanding or perhaps soft and caring, but trust that this voice will always be delivered with love.

On a daily basis, begin to act, think, and feel like the thin person you saw in your mind. Never again allow yourself to mentally see yourself as overweight. What you see in your mind is what you get in reality. Follow your Inner Visionary's advice, and go inward often to discuss your progress. Be that person from now on!

What you see in your mind is what you get in reality.

CHAPTER 5

If we really love ourselves, everything in life works.

—LOUISE L. HAY

Love Yourself Today

Practice Unconditional Self-Love, No Matter How You Are Feeling

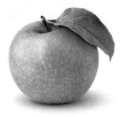

FEELINGS ARE

A PART OF YOU

THAT ARE NOT ONLY NATURAL, but are essential for self-growth and development. At the most basic level, feelings give us constant body/mind feedback about the world and any threats to our safety. They alert us to take appropriate action. At an interpersonal level, they inform us of how our relationships are serving our needs for love and support. Listening to this guidance allows us to make positive changes in our social and familial relationships. At a deeper, personal level, feelings can be our greatest motivators toward better health, career changes, and life-affirming action. All feelings, even the most painful, are powerful resources for self-discovery and wisdom.

Many of us, however, have been socially programmed to feel ashamed of having certain feelings. We have been taught that some feelings, like anger, are bad. Worse, we may have been taught that we are bad for having these feelings.

To counteract this harmful and false programming, try this self-talk technique: *"I love myself even when I feel _____."*

This will be easy when you're feeling positive emotions, because you were most likely programmed this way. But when you're experiencing negative emotions, it might be uncomfortable to be self-loving at first.

I once thought I was completely and unconditionally loving toward myself and accepting of my feelings until I tried this technique. When, while feeling upset, I said "I love myself when I feel upset" I got a twinge in my heart. This was a sure sign that my inner self didn't agree with what I had just said. I realized then and there that I had some work to do. I would have to go really deep down to love and accept myself no matter how angry, frustrated, jealous, or irritated I sometimes felt. It was a beautiful wake-up call of self-awareness.

The steps are as follows:

1. Acknowledge the feeling: i.e., *"I'm feeling angry."*

2. Say to yourself: *"I love myself even when I feel angry."*

3. How do you feel when you say that? Do you get an uncomfortable reaction from your body, mind, or emotional self? If yes, take it as a loving and valuable message that you are judging yourself harshly for having a simple feeling. Remember these basic rules about feelings: There are no bad or wrong feelings. Feelings do not define your character. They are simply temporary reactions to life events or memories.

4. Practice tuning into your feelings as they arise and say, *"I love myself even when I'm feeling_____."* If you're having trouble accepting yourself while having the feeling, repeat again the rules about feelings. With repetition, you will begin to truly accept your feelings as temporary states and you will give yourself the opportunity to fall in love with *you*.

With this simple exercise, you are changing your opinion and feelings about yourself. The more you practice this, the easier it will become. You will be permanently reprogramming yourself to experience unconditional self-love. As you let go of self-judgment, you'll find yourself less judgmental of others as well. What a wonderful benefit. It is so much better than the old standby of eating junk food!

Remember, feelings do not define you; they only reflect how you are interpreting events in the moment.

———

One way of showing love to yourself is by attaining a healthy state of mind and body. Without truly loving yourself, you run the risk of sabotaging your goals. Eating junk food and overeating are not ways of loving yourself.

— *POWER EXERCISE* —
BECOMING SELF-ACCEPTING

Here are some statements you can try out as triggers for self-judgment and criticism. If you get an emotional or physical twinge upon reading one, it's an indication that your inner self disagrees with the statement. Most likely, your Inner Critic is imposing the words "should" or "shouldn't" as a response.

Tune into the voice in your head that disagrees with each statement. It's the internal judgmental voice that is causing you to lack love and respect for yourself when you are feeling a human emotion. Examples of judgment thoughts are "I shouldn't feel angry" and "I should be happy all of the time." Once the inner voices are revealed, you are in control to change them.

I love myself even when I feel angry.

I love myself even when I feel sad.

I love myself even when I feel irritable.

I love myself even when I feel lonely.

I love myself even when I feel depressed.

I love myself even when I feel bored.

I love myself even when I feel happy.

I love myself even when I feel disgusted.

I love myself even when I feel impatient.

I love myself even when I feel weak.

I love myself even when I feel scared.

I love myself even when I feel confused.

I love myself even when I feel lazy.

I love myself even when I feel hurt.

I love myself even when I feel furious.

I love myself even when I feel successful.

I love myself even when I feel proud.

I love myself even when I feel guilty.

I love myself even when I feel insecure.

I love myself even when I feel anxious.

I love myself even when I feel shy.

I love myself even when I feel embarrassed.

I love myself even when I feel ashamed.

• Now, add your own personal statements:

"I love myself even when I feel _____."

"I love myself even when I feel _____."

"I love myself even when I feel _____."

"I love myself even when I feel _____."

> *Love yourself—accept yourself—forgive yourself—and be good to yourself, because without you the rest of us are without a source of many wonderful things.* —LEO F. BUSCAGLIA

Replace your inner critic voice with the appropriate affirmation listed above. With repetition and the intent to embrace all of your feelings as lovable parts of you, you will become more and more self-accepting. You will feel worthy to achieve your weight goals.

Repetition + Intent = YOUR KEYS TO SUCCESS

CHAPTER 6

If anything is sacred, the human body is sacred.
—WALT WHITMAN

Love Your Body Unconditionally

Thought: Do you view and treat your body as your friend or enemy?

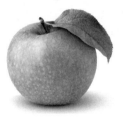

I WOULD LIKE

YOU TO BEGIN

SEEING YOUR BODY AS your best friend. After all, your body takes you where you need to go, day in and day out. It allows you the pleasures of being hugged and kissed. It is always there, loyal to the end. And, as your best friend, it deserves your love and affection.

How do you talk to and about your body? Do you ever say you hate it or that it's ugly? Would you ever talk to any of your friends that way? Would you allow your friends to speak about you in that way? Certainly not!

From this day forward, honor your body by being kind and loving toward it. When you wake up in the morning, take a few deep, slow breaths. Feel your heart beating, your lungs filling with air. Visualize a lovely day ahead, eating healthy foods, exercising, working, and playing.

QUICK TIP: When you look into the mirror, say to your body, *"I love you. Thank you for giving me life."* I suggested this tip at a presentation I gave at a Curves for Women club. I explained that it's very difficult, if not impossible, to lose weight while hating your body or yourself.

One week later, one of the women in the group, who was in her mid-sixties, approached me while I was exercising. Smiling, she told me that she started saying "I love you" to her image in the mirror and that this simple step changed her life. Like so many of us, she had given her body negative messages so often that it had become automatic. Since acknowledging her unconditional love for her body, she started to lose weight easily and, most importantly, felt happier throughout the day.

■ "HELLO, BODY. I LOVE YOU."

When you look into a mirror, do you ever say, "I'm fat"? If so, you have labeled yourself in a very painful and limiting way and will tend to live life accordingly. Overweight people overeat and eat fattening foods. They usually are lacking exercise. If you call yourself fat, you are simply programming yourself to behave in accordance with that label.

To start a new behavior you must identify yourself as a person who already lives with the new behavior. From now on, when you look into a mirror, say to yourself, *"I'm healthy, fit, and trim."* My clients initially tell me that they see this as lying. I respond by pointing out that there's a thin them inside, hidden beneath the layers of extra pounds. By saying, *"I'm healthy, fit, and trim"* you're merely acknowledging the thin person inside. And it's about time the Thin You gets acknowledged! So, it's really not a lie. It's just a shift in perspective and focus.

Here are some simple affirmations to help you connect to and love your body:

I love taking care of my body, and my body loves taking care of me.

*My body deserves my love, attention, and affection
no matter what its weight, shape, and size.*

Thank you, Dear Body, for the pleasures of life. I love you.

I am beautiful (handsome) and attractive today.

I am grateful for how my body gives me pleasure.

I treat my body like my best friend.

By saying "I'm healthy, fit, and trim," I'm acknowledging the Thin Me.

I give my body permission to lose weight and to gain strength.

I am lovable right now, just as I am.

I enjoy, honor, and respect my body.

SUCCESS JOURNAL ENTRY

Write your own affirmations of love and respect for your body, just as it is today. Start right now! Enjoy acknowledging and loving your body as your best friend.

_____

_____

_____

_____

_____

_____

_____

_____

_____

_____

_____

_____

_____

These affirmations of love will inspire you to take care of your body and to treat it with the tenderness and protection it deserves. Repeat your personal statements often, and observe how your motivation to lose weight soars!

Begin with the end in mind.
—STEPHEN COVEY

Manifesting a Healthy Body

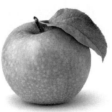

AS A HYPNO-

THERAPIST, COUNSELOR,

AND WEIGHT LOSS COACH, I've witnessed time and again the power of the mind to create, strengthen, limit, or destroy one's goals. Most of us haven't been trained how to effectively focus attention on our goals and to intentionally manifest our highest desires. Instead, most of us have been unintentionally taught to manifest the opposite of what our hearts desire by being programmed with negative expectations, thoughts, and feelings. After years of practice and disappointing results, we come to feel that not reaching our heart's goals is normal and unavoidable. We become deeply discouraged. And worse, we blame ourselves.

Manifesting is about using the power of your mind to create your life. In essence, the art of manifesting simply states that we create what we focus upon. The more attention you give a thought, negative or positive, the more strength and power it gathers.

> *To permanently lose weight, it is important*
> *to understand the power of your mind.*

Focus on your perceived limitations, and you'll feel limited. Focus on your strengths and ability to improve, and you will feel strong and able. Similarly, when you focus on how overweight you are, you can't help but continue to be overweight. I've found that growth is much easier when you learn to intentionally choose your goal, mentally focus on it, and feel it already happening and bringing you joy.

> *Realize that you, and only you,*
> *are responsible for your reality.*

Manifesting is about creating. You can manifest weight loss or weight gain. It's really up to you. I often tell my clients that they are their own hypnotherapist—that they have been unintentionally self-hypnotizing themselves to fail. I simply teach them to shift their focus and to self-hypnotize themselves to succeed.

It all begins with a goal.

Imagine you're a captain of a sailing ship, navigating through unfamiliar waters. You hold up your telescope and look for signs of land. As you turn around, you see an island that looks barren and rocky. You look in another direction and see an island that is lush and green.

As the captain, you are in control of the destination. Of course you choose the land that is life sustaining. To reach that beautiful island you must keep your vision on it and use all of the navigation tools at your disposal to keep on track. Clearly, fixing your telescope toward the rocky, barren island would make it impossible to ever reach the land of beauty and health.

Being intentional in creating the healthy body you desire begins with having a goal in mind. Intentions are created by thought, such as "150 pounds is a healthy weight for me." After establishing your goal, it's important to set it or anchor it with feeling. By setting an intention, you give it power by feeling your success already happening.

Thoughts *create* intention. Feelings *set* intention.

■ *STEP- BY-STEP MANIFESTING*

Here are the steps to manifesting the body of your dreams. Each step is equally integral to your success.

1. .**Determine Your Goal Plan.** In other words, identify where you're going so you know what path to take. For weight loss, I've found it helpful to have short-, medium- and long-term goals. This way, you'll be celebrating reaching goals often.

For most people setting short-term goals in one-pound incre- ments will make them feel successful in a short amount of time. So your first goal will be one pound less than your starting weight. Easy!

Your next short-term goal is five pounds lost.

Your mid-term goal is to reach another "decade." For example, when I weighed 165 pounds, my goal was to be in the 150s range. Then, I decided to get into the 140s, etc.

Your long-term goal is your final goal. This can be determined in a number of ways. Perhaps you remember a weight at which you felt very healthy and looked great. Feel free to use this as your long-term goal today. Remember, do not sabotage this goal with the popular myth going around today that it's impossible to reach the weight of your younger days when you're in your forties and beyond. Simply refuse to believe this limiting thought!

I am writing this book today at the age of fifty-five and am now enjoying the weight I was at in my early twenties. It is achievable. My clients and I are proof of that! How should you go about establishing a healthy weight goal for yourself? Perhaps you could seek your doctor's recom- mendation, or consult a body mass index (BMI) chart, or just let your body tell you what the right goal is.

I personally readjusted my long-term weight goal a few times during my weight loss journey. When I reached a new goal, I enjoyed being there for a while and stayed tuned into my body. After listening to my body's cues, I finally felt that being in the 120s was optimal for me. I resisted the self-sabotaging thought "that's impossible!" and fixed my focus on my new goal. Your body is your best guide.

2. **Know that you are deserving of this goal and that your good health is in the best interests of people you love and who love you.** State to yourself: "Being healthy, fit, and trim is in my highest interest and in the highest interests of all whom I love and who love me."

3. See your goal clearly, and imagine it already existing. In your heart and mind, allow no conflicting thoughts or feelings to co-exist with your goal and contaminate your vision. Use as many senses as possible.

In your mind's eye hold a mental snapshot of yourself at your goal weight, smiling, fit, and healthy. Imagine the thrill of going shopping for smaller clothes that you love. Enjoy the uplifting feelings of vibrant health, and sense your body feeling light and slender. Imagine hearing others complimenting you on how great you look.

> *The more ways you can imagine and feel your goal,*
> *the more confident and motivated you will feel.*

4. Practice, practice, practice imagining! You can do this imagining any time of the day. The more you practice, the easier it becomes. After a while, you will be able to conjure up an automatic scene in your mind at your goal weight, with all of the positive feelings and sensations automatically associated with it, instantly. In this way, you are setting and anchoring your manifestation, making it more and more powerful.

5. Hold your visualization uppermost in your mind and heart all day and night. Live with your visualization, and make it a comfortable, trusting friend. Experience and enjoy your visualization as often as possible. Be aware of any blocking thoughts, such as doubt or fear, and gently set these thoughts aside. Work at being single-minded in your view of your goal. Tell yourself, "I am free to reach my goal."

6. Make your visualization a regular part of your day. Positive visualization is akin to prayer. It gives you strength and an energetic lift. Let it inspire you to be your very best every day. Praise yourself for reaching every short-term goal, and know deeply in your heart that your long-term goal will be a reality, sooner than you think!

7. Enjoy the journey! Feel proud of yourself for having the desire and courage to take the steps for good health. Relish the joy of saying good-bye to each pound and saying hello to health and happiness. You have the power to make your weight loss journey one of joy or one of struggle. It's all in how you choose to view it.

Your mantra: *Say good-bye to each pound and say hello to health and happiness!*

THE AWESOME POWER OF ONE

One desire: *I want to be healthy.*

One thought: *I deserve this.*

One attitude: *I can do it!*

One direction: *Facing only toward your goal.*

One outcome: *Success!*

Keep your face to the sunshine and you cannot see the shadows.
—HELEN KELLER

Imagination is everything. It is the preview of life's coming attractions.

—ALBERT EINSTEIN

Mentally Rehearsing Success

What You See Is What You Get

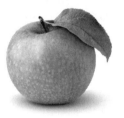

"A PINK

ELEPHANT IS

BALANCING ON A TIGHTROPE." Were you aware of an image popping into your mind when you read the previous statement? Was it perhaps of a pink elephant balancing on a tightrope?

Language provides us with instant visualization because words paint images in our minds. It's so automatic that we don't know we're doing it. If a client says, "I can't visualize," I lead them through a very simple exercise. I say, "Close your eyes and imagine a little white kitten playing with a bright red ball of yarn. Now, open your eyes and tell me what you just saw." Almost 100 percent of the time, they reply, "I saw a white kitten playing with a red ball of yarn!"

Have you ever had the experience of being in a foreign country and everyone was speaking a language you did not understand? If so, do you remember feeling frustrated? Much of the frustration comes from being unable to communicate and to get your needs met. Some of it also arises from the discomfort of lacking images in your mind. Without understanding a language, we cannot visualize. And when your mind is blank of pictures, it feels very awkward and unsettling. Visualizing is automatic, so don't worry about whether you can or can't do it. You have been visualizing ever since you learned a language! In fact, you are constantly and instantaneously visualizing as you read this book. It's impossible not to.

■ PROOF THAT VISUALIZATION WORKS

Although creative visualization, also known as "mental rehearsal," has been used by all kinds of successful people, from business executives, entrepreneurs, psychotherapists, and mastermind groups, for decades, it has been most consistently studied in the area of sports performance. Prior to the 1980 Lake Placid Olympics, a top team of Russian scientists conducted one of the most well-known studies on creative visualization in sports. In their study, four groups of Olympic athletes were compared in terms of their training schedules and performance:

- Group 1 = 100% physical training only
- Group 2 = 75% physical training with 25% mental training
- Group 3 = 50% physical training with 50% mental training
- Group 4 = 25% physical training with 75% mental training

The results were surprising. Group 4 outperformed all of the other groups!

In another classic study done by Australian psychologist Alan Richardson, three random groups of basketball players with no previous experience with visualization were selected. Each group made a series of free throws on the first and twentieth days. In the meantime, the first group practiced making free throws every day and improved 24 percent over the twenty days.

The second group had no practice and showed no improvement on the twentieth day.

The third group didn't touch a basketball for the twenty days, but were taught to visualize making free throws daily and to visualize themselves improving their aim. On the twentieth day, this group showed a 23 percent improvement; only one percentage point lower than the group that practiced daily with real balls and hoops!

These studies, and many more like them, have led experts such as Timothy Gallwye to state in his book, *The Inner Game,* "The theory of the inner game is that your performance is dependent on your state of mind. The real game is to learn how to reach that state of mind and stay in that state of mind in which your performance is best and your perception is at its clearest."

The real game for you, Reader, is to reach and hold the state of mind that will propel you to natural and permanent weight loss success!

■ *VISUALIZING AND MENTALLY REHEARSING YOUR HEALTHIEST BODY*

It takes just a small leap from the sports world to see that we can alter our ability to lose weight by focusing the mind on our desired outcome. If your self-concept has been that of an overweight person, you can change it dramatically by choosing to see yourself differently. *No image is written in stone. It is fluid.* No matter how negatively you were labeled as a child, you have the control today to change the label and, in doing so, to change your life. Only by transforming your self-image to match your desires, will you achieve life-long positive results. Hypnosis and guided imagery are powerful uses of mental rehearsal that can immediately strengthen your motivation and focus to stay on a healthy lifestyle plan.

Here is a mental rehearsal to help you imagine staying on track and losing weight. Just a few moments a day of focused attention on your goal can give you big benefits.

To begin, prepare an environment that is as conducive to relaxation as possible. Close your eyes and take a deep, cleansing breath. Feel your lungs expand with air as you breathe in. Now feel your lungs deflate like balloons emptying as you breathe out tension and stress. Set an intention to relax by saying, *"I deserve a few minutes to relax and let go."* Give your body and mind permission to take a break and to go deeply relaxed.

Notice how good it feels to allow tension and stress to melt away. Just thinking of relaxing your muscles will ease them. Imagine your muscles as warm, soft, wet noodles, so limp and loose.

Now gently focus your thoughts on your personal vision and desire for a slender, healthy body. See or imagine yourself, as though you're watching yourself on a movie screen, enjoying your day as a naturally thin person. Imagine eating small portions of healthy, life-sustaining food. You are savoring every bite, sipping water, and enjoying a slow, peaceful meal. Now imagine exercising, walking, biking, swimming. You are filled with such vital energy and heartfelt joy. You are lean, fit, and slender.

Silently say, *"What I see is what I get."*

Now see or imagine yourself losing weight. Your body is getting smaller, firmer, and healthier. Feel, with all of your senses, the success of staying healthy and thin for the rest of your life. Open your eyes when ready.

With this single-minded focus, you will succeed!

■ *ONE-MINUTE VISUALIZATIONS FOR WEIGHT LOSS*

Every thought you think automatically creates a picture in your mind, which, in turn affects your energy. *Positive pictures of success instantly generate positive energy. Negative pictures drain energy.* Quick visualizations are powerful catalysts to the life you desire. I often used these images for instant motivation during my weight loss journey and encourage you to use them or to create some that are uniquely your own.

• Visualize or imagine yourself sporting a healthy, slender body. You are smiling, feeling so happy. Notice the clothes you are wearing and how great you look wearing them.

• Imagine your friends, relatives, neighbors, and colleagues congratulating you on your weight loss. They are admiring your fit body. Notice how happy they are for your success.

• See or imagine yourself maintaining your weight loss, enjoying activities and hobbies. Shopping for new clothes is a joy, as you try on small-sized clothing. Everything in your closet fits perfectly, no matter the season.

• Visualize getting a clean bill of health at your next physical. You step on the clinic scale with pride and happiness. Your doctor is congratulating you.

- To make your visualizations more powerful, include sound, smell, and touch. For example, hear your friends saying, "You look fabulous! How did you do it? What is your secret?"

- Now imagine putting on a sleeveless top and shorts, feeling slim and healthy. *See* yourself in the mirror looking so fit and trim. *Feel* the immense pride that comes from reaching this important goal.

- Now that you're fit and trim, you enjoy fabulous baths with lovely fragrances, massages with essential oils, and shower gels with elegant scents. You love your new fit and trim body, and you love lavishing it with these fabulous smells that affirm how great you feel.

Did you get a jolt of positive energy with these quick visualizations? Create your own instant pictures of success, and feel your energy and motivation to lose weight soar!

SUCCESS JOURNAL ENTRY

Write your own customized one-minute visualizations, incorporating all five senses, for instant motivation.

_____

_____

_____

_____

_____

_____

_____

_____

_____

_____

CHAPTER 9

Sometimes affirmative beliefs are all we really need to heal us.

—HERBERT BENSON

The Power of Thought

Positive vs. Negative Affirmations

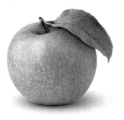

DID YOU KNOW

THAT YOU CAN

BE POSITIVELY OR NEGATIVELY affirming of yourself? You positively affirm yourself when you use statements of confidence, strength, and encouragement. Conversely, negative affirmations are messages of defeat, despair, and discouragement. Most of us have been programmed with negative thoughts that have settled into the realm of acceptance and reality. This happens because, like an endless loop of unconscious messages playing over and over again in a tape recording in our mind, they've become stuck, repeating again and again in the neural pathways of our brains. Left unexamined and unquestioned, these thoughts become a part of our belief system, which continues to perpetuate a reality that unconsciously supports our negative thinking.

Your brain is capable of generating hundreds of thoughts each minute. The thoughts to which you pay most attention form your mindset. A negative mindset, in turn, confirms and supports a predominantly unproductive inner reality in which you are viewing an internalized movie of hopelessness and failure.

I often suggest to my clients that the mind is like a computer that is being daily programmed and updated. All outside stimuli act as powerful suggestions to our subconscious minds.

> *A thought repeated enough times or that elicits a strong emotion, enters into the subconscious mind where it stays until a more positive upgrade occurs.*

■ THE POISON AND THE ANTIDOTE

Another way to think of negative affirmations is to view them as poison that seeps into your very essence, robbing you of strength and happiness. An example of a *thought poison* is when you say, *"I'll never lose the weight and keep it off."*

Positive affirmations are antidotes that neutralize the poison. When you become aware of the poisoning thought, neutralize it with the opposite. An example of an antidote to the negative affirmation, *"I'll never lose weight and keep it off,"* is *"The weight I'm losing today is permanently gone from my life."*

Each type of affirmation, negative and positive, has an opposite effect on your mood and physical strength. Negative affirmations can be huge obstacles to any plan for health and happiness.

Your thoughts create your attitude. Whether your attitude is positive or negative is entirely up to you, but either way will lead you down the emotional path that confirms and supports your thoughts. A positive attitude will strengthen you and allow you to awaken and live every day with optimism. Practicing a negative attitude will sap you of energy and make your days feel long and difficult. Furthermore, negative affirmations can actually make you physically ill while positive affirmations can increase your immunity from illness. According to Dr. Joe Dispenza, author of *Evolve Your Brain*, "Not only do our thoughts matter in how we live out our life, but our thoughts become matter right within our own body. Thoughts ... matter." *

Some fascinating studies have been done on the effects of emotions on health. One study reported in the *Journal of Advancement in Medicine* showed that changes in emotional state caused a change in an antibody that protects against illness, called S-IgA.

In this study, when participants were shown a video of Mother Theresa administering to the dying in India, feelings of compassion, love, patience, and peace were elicited. The important part was that levels of S-IgA were significantly increased as well. When the same participants felt emotions of anger, frustration, anxiety, worry, and guilt from video viewing and self-recall, their levels of S-IgA significantly dropped. This study clearly demonstrates the power of our emotions on our health.

I once gave a talk to a large group of medical professionals about the power of the mind to heal. I talked about how negative thoughts poison our lives and deplete us of energy, hope, and strength. I then suggested that the answer is simple: "If a thought is weakening you in any way, just change the thought! Practice a more positive way of viewing situations and you'll feel happier, empowered, and stronger." At the luncheon later, a woman approached me and said that when she heard that statement during the talk, she felt a wave of energy shoot up her spine. She said it was an "aha!" moment that would forever change her life. She stated it this way:

Why didn't anyone ever tell me this before? I've been struggling with down moods all of my life, and now I know that I've been caught in a cycle of negative thoughts! I never considered that I had the power or ability to simply change my thoughts. I just accepted my negative thoughts and moods as unavoidable, and something that just happened to me. How could something so simple and so obvious have been hidden from me all my life? Thank you for giving me a sense of power.

— POWER EXERCISE —

Here is a quick exercise in gaining awareness of the power of thoughts to create ability or disability. Take the time now to tune into what happens within as you slowly read the following negative statements. Sense how your mood changes with each statement. Feel your physical responses. Do these statements cause strength or weakness in you? How do your heart and stomach feel? What mental images are created? What other thoughts are elicited? It's important to do this slowly and be aware of even the tiniest of reactions.

Write down your responses to these negative statements:

• *I'm a failure. This makes me feel*

_____

_____

• *I'm fat and unattractive. This makes me feel*

_____

_____

• *Losing weight is impossible for me. This makes me feel*

_____

_____

• *Obesity runs in my family so I'm doomed to be fat. This makes me feel*

_____

_____

• *Life is too stressful. This makes me feel*

_____

_____

• *I'm lazy. This makes me feel*

_____

_____

• *I'm not good enough. This makes me feel*

_____

_____

• *I'm not smart enough. This makes me feel*

_____

_____

• *I'm too tired. This makes me feel*

_____

_____

• *I can't do it. This makes me feel*

_____

_____

• *I lack the willpower to lose weight. This makes me feel*

_____

_____

Were you able to sense how your body and feelings shifted while reading the statements? If so, did you feel yourself becoming discouraged as you read? This is a quick and easy way to witness how common and seemingly innocent statements can cause a sense of defeat in your heart, mind, and body. It doesn't even have to be your own thought. Just hearing negative statements has a huge effect on how we think and feel. When I do this exercise with my clients and workshop participants, people are amazed at how strongly and immediately their bodies react.

■ PRACTICING POSITIVE AFFIRMATIONS

One of my friends, Toni, told me how using daily affirmations allowed her to lose weight. Toni said:

Each morning while I shower I say to myself, "My cells are healthy, the healthiest they've ever been." While I say this I picture my whole body lighting up with white light energy, and that each cell in my body is light-ing up and reacting to this loving white energy. I also state, "I am healthy, happy, fit, beautiful, and full of love." One month after doing this daily routine I lost fifteen pounds, and I'm feeling wonderful.

Hypnosis is the tool I most frequently use to help my clients flood their minds, hearts, and bodies with the powerful imagery, neuro-chemistry, and emotions that support weight loss success. While they enjoy a state of deep relaxation, I saturate their subconscious minds with affirmations of effortless healthy eating and exercise, creating an inner reality of good health. In my professional experience, hypnosis is the easiest and most pleasant method of changing states of being and producing positive results. (For more information on hypnosis, please visit the appendix of this book.)

However, if you don't have access to a trained hypnotherapist, you can program your own subconscious mind with powerful affirmations for weight loss. Like my friend, Toni, you can simply repeat statements of strength and love while showering, driving, or walking. Any time you have a few minutes alone is fine.

Now it's up to you. Do you desire to feel strong, capable, and motivated during your weight loss journey? It's time to practice pow-erful self-programming that is uniquely right for you. It's time to take control of your mind and to open the door to inner strength, confi-dence, and self-love.

- The first step is to become aware of the mental chatter about you and your body.

- The second step is to make a conscious decision to change the chatter from negative to positive.

- The third step is to create a new thought pattern that empowers you.

- The final step is to practice this awareness and choice of new thoughts.

— *POWER EXERCISE* —

Tune into your physical strength, emotions, and energy levels as you read the following affirmations. Or, have someone read them to you as you relax with closed eyes. Or, better yet, record them and listen as often as you wish. Speak slowly, pausing three to five seconds between each affirmation, allowing the thought to soak into your subconscious mind. Perhaps listen during a mid-afternoon break or while falling asleep at night, programming your mind as you rest.

- *I deserve to have a healthy, slender body.*
- *I love and respect my body as my best friend.*
- *My body deserves my protection and care.*
- *I love, honor, and respect myself every day, no matter what.*
- *I handle compliments with confidence.*
- *I enjoy compliments from others.*
- *I live a life that supports good health, vitality, and self-love.*
- *I prefer to be slender rather than to overeat.*
- *Fruits and vegetables look, taste, and smell delicious.*
- *I eat in a mindful, relaxed manner.*
- *I have plenty of time to eat slowly.*
- *I enjoy leaving extra food on my plate.*
- *The more I exercise, the more I enjoy it.*
- *I am manifesting a fit, healthy, and attractive body in my life now.*
- *I am healthy today and from this day forward.*
- *I walk, talk, think, feel, and act as a healthy person.*
- *Today I'm finding clothes that look attractive on me.*
- *I have a right to say "yes" to my needs.*
- *I am eager and willing to invest the time it takes to be healthy.*
- *My optimism soars today and every day.*
- *Today is a masterpiece of my making. If I can dream it, I can do it!*
- *I am sending healing energy and love to every cell of my body.*
- *Every day, in every way, I'm getting better and better.*

Positive affirmations are statements of what you want to be true. Here are some guidelines for creating the positive statements that will powerfully affirm your weight loss success.

■ RULES FOR CREATING AFFIRMATIONS

Keep your affirmations positive. Tell yourself what you want, not what you don't want. Remember that your mind will visualize whatever you're saying and that the mind cannot see a "don't" or a "won't." Try this: tell yourself that you WON'T imagine a monkey swinging from a tree branch. I bet you saw in your mind's eye exactly what you told yourself not to see! Likewise, if you tell yourself, "I don't want to be fat," what did you just see in your mind? Remember, what you see is what you get!

1. Keep your affirmations short. This will allow your mind to get a very focused picture of your goal. It's like taking a close-up shot for a photo instead of a panoramic view of too many sights.

2. State your affirmations in the present tense. Instead of saying, "I'll be healthy someday," say "I'm healthy today."

3. Feel and enjoy the positive emotional effects of your affirmations. Emotions set your intention into place and provide the power to propel you forward. Let your heart sing with joy while feeling yourself losing weight and looking wonderfully fit and trim! This will make your weight loss journey a happy one!

4. Practice faith that what you are affirming is true. Suspend self-doubt, defeatist thoughts, and other people's negative expectations, and know that you are already successful. Share your vision with only those people in your life whom you can trust to fully support your efforts and dreams. Keep your journey as private as you wish. You cannot control what others will say and project on to you. You simply cannot afford to allow others to sabotage your dream by telling you "it's impossible."

SUCCESS JOURNAL ENTRY

*Charting your thought course will give you more power
and a fabulous record of your growth and achievement.
It will build your self-esteem and strengthen your progress
toward becoming the best that you can be.*

• *Identify a negative affirmation (venom) that has been blocking
you from losing weight. List it here:*

_____

_____

_____

_____

• *Neutralize its poisoning effect with a positive affirmation.
List it here:*

_____

_____

_____

_____

*Use your positive affirmation as a mantra to
strengthen you and to give you confidence.*

Adding more positive affirmations will build up your immunity.

Tell yourself, "I'm invincible!" Feel the power of that truth.

*Own it and enjoy it from this day forward.
And, most importantly, make it fun!*

**Remember: There is a constant conversation going on
in your head. It is what we have come to know as thinking.
Either you control it, or it controls you.**

* Dispenza, Joe, *Evolve Your Brain*, Health Communications, Inc., 2007, p 46, 187
• *Journal of Advancement in Medicine*, 1995:8(2):87–105

Beautify your thoughts. Thoughts are the headwaters of action, life, and manifestation.

—DAVID WOLFE

Counteracting Sabotaging Beliefs and Thoughts

Reprogramming for a Positive Mindset

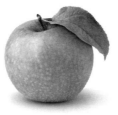

AS WE HAVE

SEEN IN THE

PREVIOUS CHAPTER, negative beliefs about our ability to lose weight not only program us to fail, they also rob us of physical strength and vitality. They can sabotage the most sincere intention to lose weight by draining us of motivation or by becoming handy excuses to fall back on when the going gets rough.

Let's go even deeper now into reprogramming our internal belief systems for weight loss success.

■ BELIEFS AND THOUGHTS THAT SABOTAGE WEIGHT LOSS SUCCESS

One of the most common sabotaging thoughts is this one: *"I'll just have one more treat and then start my diet tomorrow."* In this rationalization game, tomorrow often never comes and you lose credibility with yourself. Pretty soon, you've gained weight simply because you failed to start.

Does this scenario also sound familiar? *"I'm starting a diet tomorrow, so I might as well eat these cookies today. After all, it may be the last time I get to eat sugar for a long time."* With this mindset, you are setting yourself up for deprivation by stating and believing that all unhealthy foods are strictly off limits (diet mentality). In reality, no one can sustain 100 percent abstinence of sweets or fats. We need to be able to enjoy a piece of birthday cake now and then. The answer lies in enjoying cake now and then, not daily, and in controlling the portion size.

Some other common negative beliefs that may be sabotaging you are:

- *Healthy food is too expensive.*

- *I'm too busy to cook healthy meals.*

- *I'm too tired (upset, worried, anxious, angry) to exercise and eat healthy food today.*

- *I'll hurt the host's feelings if I don't eat the dessert.*

- *I deserve a treat today.*

- *I shouldn't waste food. I should leave an empty plate.*

Do any of these thoughts sound familiar to you? If so, it could be why you've had a hard time starting or sticking to a healthy weight loss program. Your unconscious beliefs are sabotaging you before you even begin!

You can effectively deal with these voices of despair, discouragement, and defeat by replacing them with power statements of truth.

Here are some sample statements of truth to replace the sabotage statements:

SABOTAGE STATEMENT: **Healthy food is too expensive.**
Counteract with these statements:

- *Investing in my health is a top priority to me and will pay off well into the future.*

- *I feel powerful as I budget healthy, life-affirming foods into my finances.*

- *Eating less saves me money.*

58

Conversely, if you tell yourself "I'm thin" you'll live according to that label. And no, you're not lying to yourself by saying you're thin today. The Thin You is already there. Perhaps he/she is hidden for the time being, but that part of you already exists. It's time to identify with the part of you that is thin!

New thought: "I identify with the slender, fit person that lives within me now. I love myself totally and completely."

• Co-dependency:

Old thought: "Eating is a big part of my family's get-togethers. It would be uncomfortable for them if I didn't eat Mom's cooking."

Adjustment: You can eat with your family and enjoy most of the foods that are served. Just eat smaller portions. Remember that calories do count, even on birthdays and holidays!

New thought: "My family and friends have a right to eat as they wish. I have a right to eat as I wish. I prefer that others support my weight loss efforts, but if they don't, I'll be OK. I'll still succeed. I have a right to make positive changes in my life."

• Guilt:

Old thought: "My overweight family members and friends will feel uncomfortable around me when I'm thin. I don't want them to feel bad about themselves."

Adjustment: You are not responsible for others' feelings, only for your own. See yourself as a positive role model for others wanting to lose weight. Whether someone chooses to feel inspired or intimidated by your success is up to him or her.

New thought: "I do not need outside approval from others to lose weight."

• Lack of confidence:

Old Thought: "I've failed at losing weight over and over again. I just don't have what it takes."

Adjustment: Every day is a new beginning, a new opportunity for success. The past is over, and today you have new information for successful weight loss.

New Thought: "I am learning to cope with life challenges in healthy ways. I have what it takes to be successful."

• Attachment to negative body image due to genetics:

Old Thought: "Obesity runs in my family. It's in my genes. I've always been fat and that will never change."

Adjustment: Genetics only points to predisposition, not certainty. Studies have shown that lifestyle choices can counteract genetics. If type 2 diabetes runs in your family, you are not doomed to get it. Being careful about eating sugar and starches and getting regular exercise can greatly reduce your risk of developing the disease. As Joe Dispenza says in his book, *Evolve Your Brain*, "It's true that the apple doesn't fall very far from the tree, but that doesn't mean that it can't roll to another location." *

New Thought: "Regardless of what I've weighed in the past or now weigh, I can choose to weigh less and confidently act on that choice. Genetics is only one part of the total picture. The most important part of the picture is lifestyle choices. I can take 100 percent control of those choices."

• Diet Mentality:

Old Thought: "Dieting is painful and difficult, and leads to failure."

Adjustment: You are not on a diet, but are making important positive lifestyle changes that will lead to permanent weight loss. These new ways of eating will soon become your "new normal" and will be automatic and easy.

New Thought: "I am choosing a healthy eating and exercise plan that is permanent and life-affirming. The joy I get in losing weight and looking wonderful will keep me motivated to maintain my perfect weight and fitness forever."

• Exhaustion:

Old Thought: "I hate to exercise and cooking healthy foods is too time consuming. I'm too tired at the end of the day."

Adjustment: Leading a sedentary life causes sluggishness and apathy, while being active stimulates energy. As difficult as it might be to start, try to exercise a little every day. At first you may have to force yourself to exercise when you're tired, but chances are that you'll feel renewed by it. Resist the urge to lie on the couch after eating dinner. Instead, take a little walk. Get interested in cooking healthy meals by finding and trying new recipes. Steaming vegetables doesn't take much longer than going through a fast food drive-through or making a prepackaged meal.

New Thought: "Cooking healthy meals is a pleasurable way of taking care of my body. Exercise is my favorite stress releaser and is a highlight of my day! My health is my top priority."

Imagine yourself as an archer, aiming at the target (your goal weight). If you say to yourself, *"This is futile. I'll never lose the weight,"* your bow is essentially pointed at the ground and your arrow will hit the dirt over and over again. If, instead, you see yourself as an archer with bow in perfect alignment for shooting a straight arrow, right on target, you are creating a thought pattern for success. When you set your sights only on the target, focus directly on your abilities and strength, and practice only thoughts of success ... then you will succeed.

* Dispenza, Joe, *Evolve Your Brain*, Health Communications, Inc., 2007. p 187

CHAPTER 11

You are a child of the universe, no less than the trees
or the stars. You have a right to be here.
—FROM *DESIDERATA*

Letting Go of Toxic Shame that Binds Us to Failure

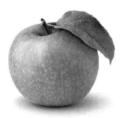

LIKE MANY OF

YOU, MY WEIGHT

CREPT UP OVER THE YEARS. I was in severe denial of how out of shape I was until one day I saw a photograph of a person I didn't recognize. That person was me! This revelation, as painful as it was, gave me a gift. Its gift was the power to break through the wall called denial. I couldn't lie to myself any longer and get away with it. I saw the truth.

I have to tell you, I had to practice some major self-forgiveness at that moment before I could feel strong, focused, and deserving of a slender body. I had to heal from a deep-seated feeling of shame that I felt about gaining so much weight.

Shame is a powerful negative force, which can sabotage any success plan you may make. Some of us grew up feeling huge guilt when we made even the most minor of mistakes and have internalized that emotion. No matter how unfair, society also points the painful finger of Shame and its brother, Blame, at people who are overweight.

■ WHAT IS TOXIC SHAME?

Toxic shame is an internalized self-identity that makes us believe we are flawed, bad, and inadequate. Like most belief systems, it is often established early in childhood well before we are able to use critical thinking.

This happens when a parent says to a child "shame on you" or embarrasses the child, or reacts to a child's behavior with a look of disgust or with sarcasm. It happens when a child is crying and a parent shouts, "stop crying!" or "stop being such a baby!" It happens when a child's feelings get discounted, disregarded, ignored, or criticized. It creates within the child a deep sense of abandonment and unworthiness.

As a licensed parent educator, I taught parenting classes for thirteen years. In my classes, I explained that it's appropriate for parents to label their child's behavior, but not appropriate to label the child's character. By labeling a child "bad boy "or "bad girl," you are locking him or her in a box called "inadequate."

Instead of simply seeing that she has made a mistake, the child feels like she is a mistake. Shame-based parenting can create a very wounded child who tries to please everyone but herself. The idea within the mind and heart of the child becomes: "If I can just be perfect and good enough, Mommy and Daddy will finally love me."

But the truth is that perfection is impossible, and therefore, this child never feels, deep down, like a good or worthy person. This is disabling in many ways because a person who feels fundamentally flawed is less able to make self-respecting and self-loving choices and will try to fill the void with outside approval or love. Sometimes this love comes from food. Food, after all, never disapproves of or disrespects us. Food can feel very, very safe.

The comforting news is that you can release the wounding childhood programming that has continued to harm and weaken you, and this book will show you how.

Internalized toxic shame keeps us locked in a prison cell of low self-worth. Trapped within this prison cell, we feel a hopeless sense of despair and emptiness. We feel powerless to be in control of our destiny. We feel intrinsically unlovable, inadequate, and lonely.

Can a person who feels fundamentally flawed, worthless, and inadequate ever be able to truly love himself or herself and feel worthy of a healthy body? I believe this is one of the main reasons why people "fail" at diets. They simply don't feel worthy or capable of succeeding. The good news is this: Yes! A person who feels fundamentally flawed absolutely can change! She can learn to love herself and to feel worthy of a healthy body. My clients are doing it every day, and I can help you do the same.

■ *THE PERFECTIONISM / SHAME LOOP*

People who come from a shame-based family often develop a ruthless sense of perfectionism. In shame-based families, actions and feelings are either right or wrong. There are no gray areas, and there's no room for mistakes. If you did something that is believed to be wrong by the family, you are wrong as a person. In a shame-based family, the words "should" and "shouldn't" are freely and often used. These words say "shame on you for making a mistake." They define you as a flawed person.

What does this have to do with losing weight? If you have internalized a shame-based personality, you may find yourself saying things like "I shouldn't have eaten that piece of cake" or "I should exercise more." You feel like a bad person every time you let yourself down. Armed with the judgment words of "should" and "shouldn't," the internalized voice of your Inner Critic harshly and unfairly continues to judge your character as "bad."

■ *THE LOOP OF JUDGMENT*

Within this perfectionist mindset, you are either good or bad. You are either on or off a diet. When you're following the diet rules, you feel like a good person. When you break a diet rule, you feel like a bad person. Feeling like a bad person triggers inner shame and can often cause us to turn to food for comfort, thereby numbing our negative emotions. Toxic shame statements, like the following two, are so intense with self-loathing that they actually fuel addictive behavior.

I am a worthless human being.

I am unlovable and unattractive because I'm overweight.

Statements like these create feelings that are overwhelming and unbearable. They make us feel hopeless, and this sense of hopelessness feeds despair and depression. This is how food becomes a loyal friend, always there for us. Food never abandons us or tells us we are bad. Food tastes good and seems to fill the void in our heart. Over time, we learn to reach for food to numb, bury, or cover up our self-disgust.

A shame-based person feels so vulnerable that she has difficulty dealing with criticism. Even a slight overture of criticism or rejection can send her to the refrigerator, reaching for her best friend: food. How can you stop this reaction to criticism? Realize that when someone criticizes you, it says absolutely nothing about *you*. It is simply that person expressing his or her thoughts, perceptions, and feelings in that moment. Their judgment of you only defines them as a person who is choosing to behave in a critical, judgmental way. It does not define you in any shape, form, or fashion.

Hugh Prather in his book, *Notes to Myself*, makes this attitude changing aha! discovery by realizing:

> *Before, I thought I was actually fighting for my own self-worth; that is why I so desperately wanted people to like me. I thought their liking me was a comment on me, but it was a comment on them. The question I could ask myself after receiving criticism is "does his statement give me any insights into myself," not "is it true?"*

Feelings are not right or wrong. They are our allies. Your feelings deserve to be heard, felt, and respected. You don't need to act on all feelings. Just acknowledge them and ask, *"What is the message this feeling is giving to me?"* and *"How is this feeling giving me an opportunity to grow and learn?"* Remember, feelings hurt most when they are discounted or ignored. Embrace them as a loving part of you.

Have you internalized statements of shame for gaining weight? If so, are you ready to release them and embrace self-love and forgiveness? Remember, you are an awesome human being, worthy of happiness, love, and good health TODAY.

First, go inward and identify any statements of shame that you may have absorbed through the years. Once you identify them, they are no longer hidden from your consciousness. Once revealed, you have the power to face them and dissolve them. Statements of shame are those that make you feel like a bad or unworthy person. They are the inner statements that make you feel unlovable and undeserving. Left unquestioned and unchallenged, they even have the power to make you feel unattractive, unimportant, and less-than.

Shaming statements about weight are:

• *I should have lost weight by now.*

• *I'm the fat one in the family.*

• *I shouldn't buy new clothes because I look so fat.*

• *I'm ugly.*

• *I'm a loser. I can't stay on a diet.*

• *I'm hopeless and weak. I should be stronger.*

• *I shouldn't even try to lose weight. I can't stick with it.*

You cannot change how you were raised, but you can change how you treat yourself today. The past is over. Your true power lies in the Now.

■ *BANISHING SHAME PERMANENTLY*

An article written for *Science News* (April 24, 2010) reported a study done in which people were asked to write down a memory of a bad decision they had made. Half the participants handed their notes directly to the experimenter and the other half first put the note into an envelope before turning them in. Interestingly, those who had sealed their painful memory into the envelope felt fewer negative feelings about themselves afterward than those who only handed the paper to the experimenter.

Using the results of this study, let's "seal and give away" any negative messages you may have internalized about your body shape, size, and weight.

Take a moment to think about any shaming messages you have internalized about your weight. When do you "should" yourself into a dark, lonely pit of hopelessness and inadequacy? Write these messages on a piece of paper. Take your time to come up with your list.

When you are ready to release these statements say, *"I acknowledge that these statements are false, and therefore, I release them from my identity, today and from this day forward."*

Now, symbolically let go of the harmful messages. You may wish to tear the paper up as you feel an emotional commitment to truly let go of the shame. Or, if you prefer, put the paper into a shredder or into a fire. Or perhaps, like the study participants, you choose to seal the messages inside an envelope and give the envelope to someone and walk away.

Whatever way you choose to symbolically remove the shame messages, feel how great it feels to be released from untrue, painful statements!

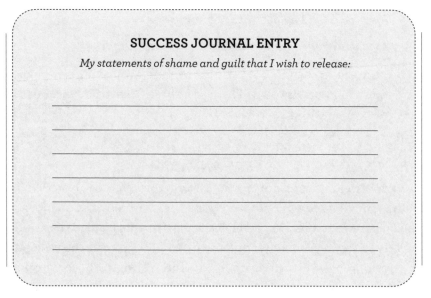

SUCCESS JOURNAL ENTRY

My statements of shame and guilt that I wish to release:

Release these statements in any symbolic way that feels right to you. Get rid of them!

Now, build a sense of power, acceptance, and love by repeating the following statements. Feel free to write these on a piece of paper and read them often until they become internalized. Add your own statements of self-acceptance and self-worth.

Today I am reclaiming my birthright of personal power.

Today I am committed to loving myself just as I am.

I am uniquely ME.

I have purpose and value, no matter what size or weight I am.

I have willpower.

I trust myself to make positive, healthy choices in eating.

I am worthy of success.

Others' opinions of me do not define who I am. I define who I am.

My definition of myself is flexible and open for revision,
but always loving and kind.

I have a right to make mistakes and learn from them.

I deserve to be treated with respect.

My needs are important.

My feelings are my allies.

I am proud of who I am.

SUCCESS JOURNAL ENTRY

Write your own unique statements of worth and power:

_____

_____

_____

_____

_____

CONGRATULATIONS ON HAVING THE
COURAGE TO ACCEPT ALL PARTS OF YOU!

■ *THE NEXT STEP: FORGIVENESS*

By releasing the toxic shame that binds us to failure, we can take the next important step to emotional freedom: forgiveness.

It's time to fully forgive yourself and others and to move steadfastly forward.

Affirmations for Forgiveness

- *Today, and from this day forward, I forgive myself for eating in unhealthy ways.*

- *Today, and from this day forward, I forgive others and myself for shaming me in any way regarding my weight.*

- *Today, and from this day forward, I forgive anything that I, or anyone else, did in my past that led to my weight gain.*

- *The past is over. I am making life-changing decisions today that are allowing me to reach my weight loss goals, once and for all.*

- *I do the best I can every day. I let go of expectations of perfection and celebrate my commitment to change.*

SUCCESS JOURNAL ENTRY

Write your own statements of forgiveness:

_____

_____

_____

_____

_____

_____

_____

_____

When I was fourteen my class had to write a home essay on
ourselves. Mine began: "Time lies heavily on my hands."
My parents were upset by this because they said it reflected
on them. "You always have plenty to do ... and it shows how
ungrateful you are for all we have done for you."
So I changed the opening to "I find life full of interest."
They were happy, and I got a "Very Good."
— R. D. LAING

CHAPTER 12

When I let go of what I am, I become what I might be.
—LAO TZU

Fran's Success Story

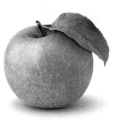

FRAN WAS A SINGLE,

THIRTY-YEAR-OLD

CORPORATE ACCOUNTANT WHO was desperate to lose weight. She was almost 80 pounds overweight and her confidence had hit rock bottom. She was tired of failing at crash diets. Fran came to me and said, "You are my last resort. This *has* to work!"

When I asked why she so badly wanted to lose weight, she replied that she was tired of watching her colleagues climb the ladder of success while she was overlooked time and time again. Fran wondered out loud if her weight was hindering her from being promoted and from making friends.

It was apparent that this was a very lonely young woman who needed help discovering her inner beauty and strength. Exploring further, Fran began to realize that she, like many of us, had habitually turned to food when life got difficult. In other words, she was an emotional eater.

I explained to her that without learning how to emotionally cope with life's difficulties, diets simply would not work for long. I first helped Fran think about and state her personal goals, as well as discuss any inner blocks that were restricting her from reaching these goals.

One block, Fran told me, was that she never really learned how to deal with emotions in healthy ways. These are her words:

> I was a latchkey kid. My parents each worked sixty-hour weeks and were worn out and stressed out much of the time. They had their cocktail hour every evening while waiting for the take out delivery boy to arrive. There were frequent fights between my parents, and I remember feeling frightened and alone a lot. I discovered at an early age how to soothe myself with food. I hid food in my bedroom and forgot all of my problems as I snacked after school on candy and chips. Eating alone in my bedroom was my special time of relaxation throughout childhood. Also, I was expected to be the perfect daughter. I still regard failures as crises, and I absolutely panic when I make mistakes. The impossibility of being perfect all the time makes me want to give up and do nothing.

■ FRAN'S STEPS TO HEALING

I reminded Fran that she was not responsible for what she did and did not learn in childhood, but that she was responsible for the way she lived her life today. I assured her that she could retrain herself to deal with emotions without food and that she could accomplish her goals with confidence and strength. I then showed her how to write affirmations to reflect her goals and to dissolve her emotional blocks. I also suggested she journal her statements and progress. Hypnosis allowed her to experience, on a deeply emotional level, the achievement of her goals as though they were already accomplished. Under hypnosis, Fran was guided to envision her body as healthy and attractive. She was led to feel the happiness of being active and in control of her feelings and eating habits.

Positive post-hypnotic suggestions for continued motivation and success were added before she was guided to return to full consciousness. Upon opening her eyes, Fran felt rejuvenated and optimistic about losing weight. She said she just couldn't believe how deeply relaxed she felt and how eager she was to continue her program.

She decided to enjoy the deeply relaxing benefits of my *Weight Loss Hypnosis* CD after work, instead of guiltily snacking on junk food. Combining hypnosis with her own work of affirming and visualizing her goals between sessions, Fran was able to stay motivated and happy throughout her weight loss program. She got out more, established friendships, and confidently applied for job promotions. In the process, she lost the eighty pounds while her self-esteem and self-respect soared!

Fran's personal statements, listed below, are wonderful examples of how to state goals clearly and how to keep thoughts in the positive. She has generously given me permission to share them with anyone who may find them useful as guides in his or her weight loss journey. Notice how although Fran's main goal in coming to see me was to lose weight, not all of her stated goals and affirmations are about eating. In fact, you will see that most of her statements never mention food, but instead refer to her emotions, life vision, and desires.

Losing weight is not just about the food you eat, but more importantly it is about how you feel about yourself and how you deal with life's challenges.

■ FRAN'S AFFIRMATION STATEMENTS

What I want:
- *To lose and maintain a healthy weight.*
- *To feel good about my body.*
- *To enjoy hobbies: music, traveling, gardening, biking.*
- *To feel comfortable trying new things.*
- *To start dealing with physical and emotional stress without eating.*
- *To nurture a positive attitude.*

Affirmations that support my desires:
- *I am healthy.*
- *I am perfect just the way I am.*

- *I am able to cope with my emotions in healthy ways.*
- *I am able to deal with fear.*
- *I am able to deal with disappointment.*
- *I am able to deal with responsibility.*
- *I stay calm under stress.*
- *I live in the present.*
- *I feel comfortable with who I am.*
- *I am able to accomplish anything I set out to do.*
- *I have the ability to change.*
- *I have an appetite for healthy food.*
- *I eat only healthy food when I'm under stress.*
- *I forgive myself when I feel afraid.*
- *I am enthusiastic about my life.*
- *I feel motivated to accomplish my goals.*
- *I counterbalance any negative with a positive.*
- *I have the ability to put my goals into action.*
- *By staying active in life, I keep my mind and body healthy.*
- *I am able to express emotions as they come.*
- *Positive action is my new habit for the rest of my life.*
- *I feel comfortable around large groups of people.*
- *I eat in healthy ways when I'm in large groups of people.*
- *I enjoy being in a loving relationship.*
- *Failures are steppingstones to better things.*
- *Strength, learning, and knowledge come from mistakes.*
- *I am strong today.*

SUCCESS JOURNAL ENTRY

Write your goal statements (What I Want). Do it now ... Don't wait!

_____

_____

_____

_____

_____

_____

_____

_____

Write the affirmations that will support your goals:

_____

_____

_____

_____

_____

_____

_____

_____

_____

_____

By using your own affirmations that reflect your desires, you will have an inner support system that will motivate you to success!

CHAPTER 13

Our lives are not determined by what happens to us but by how we react to what happens, not by what life brings to us, but by the attitude we bring to life. A positive attitude causes a chain reaction of positive thoughts, events and outcomes. It is a catalyst, a spark that creates extraordinary results. —ANONYMOUS

Dealing with Emotions without Eating

Experts today estimate that at least 75 percent of overeating is triggered by emotions.

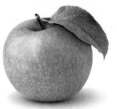

EVERY LIFE HAS ITS SHARE OF SADNESS, FRUSTRATION, and anger as well as joy and happiness. These are normal human emotions. If, like many people, you reach for food in response to feelings, you can begin to deal with emotions in healthier ways:

- **Practice** looking for evidence that you are not a victim of life's events, and instead begin to take personal responsibility for your reactions.

- **Consider** how sadness and disappointment are really gifts that offer priceless opportunities to become wiser, more empathetic, and stronger.

- **Witness** the patterns that show up in your life, and choose to react in different and healthier ways to the patterns. Notice how each pattern dissolves when you no longer respond in ineffective and predictable ways.

Remember, you are not in control of how others choose to treat you, but you are in control of your responses. It's time to choose healthy responses!

■ *DEALING WITH STRESS WITHOUT EATING*

To take eating out of your stress management plan, you need a new plan that offers healthy ways of dealing with life's challenging events. And of course, the best action is one of prevention. Just as it's beneficial to build up a strong immune system by regularly eating healthy food and taking supplements, it's in your best interest to also build stress immunity. Becoming more stress immune will give you the ability to withstand crisis with greater mental clarity and emotional strength. Don't wait for a crisis to occur before you begin meditating or before you begin practicing relaxation skills. Start a practice now to build your inner defense system of coping skills.

Here are some simple ways to prevent and deal with life stress:

1. Rename the word "stress." Are you in the habit of describing a day that is busy and filled with commitments as "stressful"? If so, remember that just saying to yourself or out loud, "I'm so stressed!" causes dangerous stress hormones to flow and, if repeated often, creates a habitual state of anxiety. I often suggest to my clients to stop using the word "stress" for a week or so, replace the stress statements with coping statements and to notice any attitudinal and physical changes that result. For instance, many of my clients enjoy replacing the old stress statement with this one: "I am having a busy day, and I love being busy!" With this new way of labeling their days, they often begin to see and appreciate the opportunities for growth and productivity that an activity-filled life brings. And in doing so, they can enjoy new habitual feelings of gratitude and excitement, instead of dread and tension. Remember, all events are neutral until you assign them meaning. The meaning you give an event gives it the power to create your feeling state when the event occurs.

• *My stress statement replacement is:*

_____

_____

_____

_____

2. Sweat out the stress with exercise. Exercise increases feel-good endorphins, lowers cortisol, and promotes restful sleep. When you feel stress beginning to build up, get some exercise and feel the stress melt away!

• *When I feel stressed, I will move my body in these ways:*

_____

_____

3. Boost your "Vitamin C" (as in Connection). One of the main characteristics of people who live long and healthy lives is that they have a strong social support system. Just getting out of the house and mingling with others will give you a sense of community and connection.

• *Ways I will now frequently connect with others:*

_____

_____

4. Enjoy pets and nature. Studies have shown a significant reduction in blood pressure when people pet cats or dogs. And the pets love it as well! Connecting with pets allows you to enter their quiet world of simplicity, unconditional love, and present moment existence. I brush my cat, Agate, every night as a little ritual she and I both enjoy. Listening to her purr and watching her close her eyes in response to the brush strokes makes me instantly feel more relaxed and, at least for the time being, unencumbered by the day's concerns and problems. If you don't have a pet, sit by a window and observe the outside animals. I have a large maple tree in my front yard and one of my favorite activities is to lie on the couch watching the birds and squirrels make a home for themselves in the large branches. They're quite comical to watch. I also love observing how the tree changes with the seasons. Even in the winter it is beautiful in its simplicity.

In addition, becoming more intimate with nature can be a wonderful daily meditation and a way to comfort yourself during a stressful day. When I walk around the lake in my neighborhood, I take care to observe my thoughts and try to gently release stressful, negative thoughts that might damage my body and emotions. I look for the dogs and their owners who frequent the lake walk. I look at signs of the seasons changing, of the day beginning or ending. I walk in silent meditation within the safety and beauty of nature.

How I will now enjoy nature to reduce stress:

_____

_____

These steps for dealing with stress are just the beginning. Now look for other ways to deal with everyday stress without eating. If you are having difficulty, perhaps observe how the thin people in your life handle stress and make their healthy responses part of your plan.

My commitment statements:

My new ways of dealing with stress are:

_____

_____

Mentally rehearse these, and notice how great it feels to take positive action.

■ DEALING WITH LONELINESS WITHOUT EATING

Do you ever think of food as a best friend? If so, keep in mind this truth: *Food is nothing more than an inanimate object. It can never replace human interaction and love.* If, at the moment, you are feeling a lack of loving relationships in your life, seek counseling or take positive action to meet new friends. Sitting in front of your TV while eating junk food is completely counterproductive to your desire for meeting new people. A potential best friend or spouse cannot even meet you if you're secluded in your home eating night after night.

I once read a quote that said, "To make friends, be friendly." I like the simplicity of that thought. Let's first talk about being friendly with the person who never, ever leaves you: *yourself!*

Always remember that you are never truly alone when you discover that you have a built-in relationship with yourself. What is your dialogue with *you*? Are you friendly, loving, and nonjudgmental with yourself? Many of us seek approval and love from outside relationships without first developing a healthy relationship within. When you talk to yourself in friendly, optimistic ways about yourself and the world, you become less dependent upon others to provide that for you. You begin to feel more and more comfortable spending time alone, and effortlessly move from being with others to being alone. You no longer fear solitude. I can't tell you how liberating this is!

The first step is to develop a loving relationship with yourself, which is a main objective of this book. Decide to nurture the truth that you deserve to be treated in respectful and loving ways. Be that person in your life, first and foremost. Then, and only then, will you attract others who will treat you with love and respect. When you understand that we attract mirror images of our inner selves, you realize it all starts with *you*.

Of course, even people who have developed healthy relationships with themselves feel a need for companionship. We are social beings after all. When you are lonely for companionship, consider and practice reactions such as these before reaching for food:

- *Play with a pet.*
- *Participate in a spiritual community of your choice.*
- *Join a sports league.*
- *Volunteer at a hospital or school.*
- *Take a night course in something that interests you.*
- *Go to a public place (museum, park, theater, library, café), and become a people-watcher. Smile and say hello to strangers you meet at public places. It makes everyone feel more connected and lifts depression. In other words, be friendly!*
- *Cultivate a new friendship with a neighbor or with a work colleague. Take responsibility for taking the first step!*
- *Mentor a child (grandchild, niece, nephew, neighbor's child).*

• *Sign up for a gym membership, and use it every week.*

• *Add your own:*

_____

_____

_____

_____

My commitment statement:

When I feel lonely, I will:

_____

_____

_____

_____

Mentally rehearse these, and notice how great it feels to take positive action.

Other emotions that commonly lead us to overeat are anger and boredom. Here are samples of healthy alternatives to these emotions.

■ DEALING WITH ANGER WITHOUT EATING

• *Run around the block.*

• *Scream into a pillow.*

• *Cry.*

• *Write a letter to the person who is angering you. Don't mail it.*

• *Turn on loud music and dance!*

• *Take a car ride. Shout your feelings out loud, or sing to loud music on the radio.*

• *Phone an understanding friend, and share your feelings.*

• Add your own:

_____

_____

_____

My commitment statement:

When I feel angry, I will:

_____

_____

_____

_____

Mentally rehearse these, and notice how great it feels to take positive action.

■ DEALING WITH BOREDOM WITHOUT EATING

Activities or hobbies I enjoy are:

_____

_____

_____

_____

When I feel bored, I will:

_____

_____

_____

_____

Mentally rehearse these, and notice how great it feels to take positive action.

■ *MY PLAN FOR DEALING WITH ALL EMOTIONS WITHOUT EATING:*

Of course, there are many emotions other than stress, loneliness, boredom, and anger that can trigger a habitual eating response. Remember that the only appropriate time for eating is when you are physically hungry.

Make a list of how you will now respond to everyday emotions without reaching for food.

- *When I feel frustrated, I now choose to* _____

- *When I feel sad, I now choose to* _____

- *When I feel happy, I now choose to* _____

- *When I feel like celebrating, I now choose to* _____ ____

- *When I feel confused, I now choose to* _____

- *When I feel anxious, I now choose to* _____

- *When I feel relaxed, I now choose to* _____

- *When I feel depressed, I now choose to* _____

- *When I feel tired, I now choose to* _____

What other emotions trigger you to eat? Add them to your list:

- *When I feel* _____ *, I now choose to* _____

- *When I feel* _____ *, I now choose to* _____

- *When I feel* _____ *, I now choose to* _____

- *When I feel* _____ *, I now choose to* _____

- *When I feel* _____ *, I now choose to* _____

Mentally rehearse these, and notice how great it feels to take positive action.

Keep your lists handy for easy reference. Now that eating is no longer your "go to" reaction to emotions, you will automatically consume fewer calories and enjoy greater life balance and satisfaction. As you practice your new healthy behavior, the pounds will effortlessly melt away!

CHAPTER 14

The greatest thing we can do is let people know
that they are loved and capable of loving.
—FRED ROGERS

The Strength of a Support System

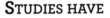

STUDIES HAVE

NOT ONLY CONFIRMED

THE STRONG LINK OF lasting weight loss and interpersonal support, but show that the more social support you receive, the more weight you are prone to lose and keep off.*

As is true in making any new changes in life, it's beneficial to have at least one person who can act as your coach and motivator. For some, it's a trusted therapist or personal trainer. For others, it's a friend or work colleague. For me, a main support system during my weight loss journey was my sister, Janice. Unconditionally loving, Janice has the incredible gift of being able to be honest without being harsh or critical.

When I was at my heaviest, she never judged me. When I was in total denial, she was kind and unconditionally respectful. When I simply wasn't in the correct place of consciousness to make drastic changes in my eating lifestyle, she gently reminded me that I used to be healthier and thinner.

I remember she once said, "I think your main problem is that you need more muscle toning." This got me thinking about starting to exercise and led me to join Curves for Women. Curves is an emotionally safe place, especially for overweight women who may feel intimidated in a mixed gender gym. Women of all ages, shapes, and sizes belong to my Curves location, and several of them have become a mini-support group for fitness. We encourage each other and notice when one of us has lost weight. We share nutrition tips and healthy recipes. I am confident that an organization similar to Curves exists almost everywhere.

One of my favorite Curves members is Vivian Hempel. Vivian, who recently turned 98-years-old, shows up regularly for exercise sessions and keeps up with the fast pace of the 30-second circuit stations. She even routinely ends her exercise time with several minutes of hula-hoop! She's an amazing example of how just a little bit of time and effort pays off in a very big way in determining our quality of life. Vivian doesn't let the negative myths of aging deter her. She still identifies herself as a vital, vibrant, and interesting woman.

Another inspirational woman in my life is my mother, Vivian Volk. My mom gave birth to four sets of twins and one single child, within eight years. Each pregnancy reached full term! Even with the twin pregnancies and the stress of raising nine children, Mom never had a weight issue. Today, at age 85, Mom is slender and fit, enjoying her retirement community in New Jersey while frequently walking, biking, and attending dances and exercise classes. For added recreation, Mom plays the organ and sings beautifully. She is a loving role model of how to age with grace and beauty. Thank you, Mom!

Another support is my friend, Kris Nelson, whom I lovingly refer to as my "personal health guru." Kris, who is a vivacious, energetic 64-year-old, keeps up-to-date with sound nutrition facts and is always available for a walk, regardless of weather conditions. We also enjoy healthy food shopping and cooking together. She is kind and encouraging, and I deeply value her friendship and healthy lifestyle support.

■ MARTHA AND GENE

My clients, Martha and Gene, married for 35 years, had each slowly gained an extra fifty pounds over the years. I suggested that they become each other's weight loss support person, and together we came up with a plan that would fit their interests and lifestyle. They now begin each day with an early morning workout at the gym before work. They plan, shop for, and cook healthy meals together, relax to my *Weight Loss Hypnosis* CD after work, and take a walk after dinner. Not only have they lost weight together, but they have also renewed a beautiful closeness in their relationship. As Martha recently told me, "Instead of sitting in front of the TV all night, snacking on junk food, we are having fun losing weight. This is a lifestyle change that we can definitely stick with."

Who is your support system? Of course, mention yourself as the primary support. Be your own inner coach and admirer. Praise yourself for any and all healthy changes you've made, no matter how small. Set weight loss goals, and visualize yourself attaining those goals. Cheer yourself with every step you take on your path to health!

Next, find someone in your life who cares about you and whom you trust will support your efforts. Think who that might be. For some people, it might even be a deceased relative who had been unconditionally loving in life. Think about that person in spirit, cheering you on and loving that you're making strides toward a better life.

■ BUILDING YOUR SUPPORT

1. Think about a person in your life who has unconditionally loved and supported you. Think about that person now. Feel their encouraging and supportive energy flow into you and within you. Let their loving energy inspire and strengthen you all day.

2. Think of someone you know and like who also wants to lose weight. Ask if he or she would like to take walks or attend a gym with you. Perhaps you decide to meet at one another's home and exercise together with a DVD.

Janice and I live 2,000 miles apart; she is in New Jersey and I am in Minnesota. When we want to lose a few pounds, we start up our Scale Club. We weigh in every Tuesday morning and report to each other. Sometimes we have other friends and relatives join in. This gives us accountability and support, and it's free! We also bike once a week on our stationary bikes while watching a favorite TV show and call each other on the phone during commercials. We have found something that works for us and is fun. What would work for you? Start today and enjoy the re-wards of taking positive action toward reaching your weight loss goals!

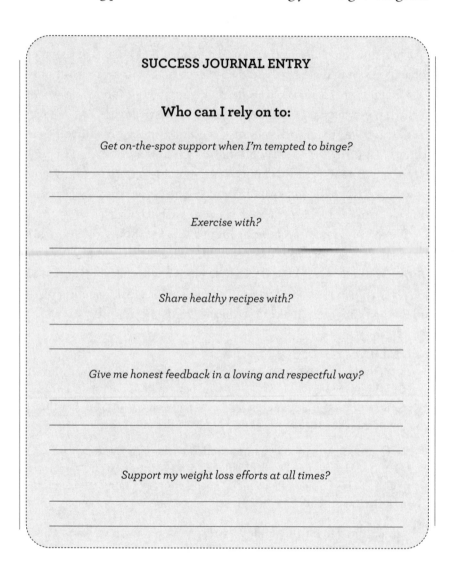

SUCCESS JOURNAL ENTRY

Who can I rely on to:

Get on-the-spot support when I'm tempted to binge?

_____

_____

Exercise with?

_____

_____

Share healthy recipes with?

_____

_____

Give me honest feedback in a loving and respectful way?

_____

_____

Support my weight loss efforts at all times?

_____

_____

Wing R.R. and Jeffery R.W., Benefits of Recruiting Participants with Friends and Increasing Social Support for Weight Loss and Maintenance. *J Consult Clin Psychology.* 1999 Feb. 67 (1): 132-38.

Christakis N.A. and Fowler J.H., The Spread of Obesity in a Large Social Network Over 32 Years. *The New England Journal of Medicine.* 2007 July: 357 (4): 370-79.

CHAPTER 15

*You gain strength, courage and confidence by every experience in
which you really stop to look fear in the face ... You must do the thing
you think you cannot do.* —ELEANOR ROOSEVELT

Healthy Eating During Times of Crisis

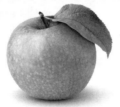

AS I WRITE

THIS CHAPTER,

I AM REFLECTING on the multitude of global hardships and crises
that have occurred in the past several years. We recently witnessed one
of the greatest stock market crashes in history, a crash that has defined
these times as "The Great Recession."

Shock, anger, and confusion were palpable as our life savings
dissolved in front of our eyes. Panic. Waiting for the recovery that never
seems to come, things have become even more precarious as homes are
in foreclosure, jobs are lost, and spilled oil continues to flow into our
oceans and beaches, killing the most vulnerable and innocent amongst
us: wildlife. Horrified, we are now constantly looking over our shoul-
ders, bracing for the next crisis, while trying to deal with a persistent
sense of despair and hopelessness. Without our knowledge, we often seem
to slip into a defensive panic mode. It can be helpful to understand exactly
what is happening.

■ *THE EMOTIONAL BRAIN*

As humans, we benefit from a highly evolved brain. The older portion of our brain we might call our emotional brain. Over the entire

history of our species, our emotional brain has enabled us to recognize life-threatening situations and to take reflexive action to keep us alive. This is the oft-mentioned "fight or flight" response. It is instinctual, automatic, and beneath the level of consciousness.

In situations of primitive survival, there was no time to think. There was only time to act. There is no thinking involved with our emotional brain. When our ancient ancestors met up with a saber-toothed tiger at a watering hole on the savannah, they either acted or were eaten.

The fact that you are here today reading this text would indicate that your ancestors had sensitive emotional brains that kept them alive to breed. They were more prepared to recognize danger and respond by fleeing or fighting. Back in our history, this was clearly a great blessing. However, with every blessing, a curse may exist and cause us more harm than good.

■ *THE THINKING BRAIN*

The much newer and more highly developed portion of our brain, the thinking brain, is capable of dealing with much more complex reasoning. This is the wondrous ability that separates humans from the rest of their fellow creatures. The thinking brain is capable of confronting highly complex issues and analyzing them through reason and logic to creatively improve our lives. Almost all of the benefits of modern living, starting with the wheel and moving all the way to space travel, are made possible through the thinking brain. Today, most of our brain mass is made up of this newer thinking brain.

Brain research over the last thirty years has brought us to a point where we can begin to understand the dynamic interplay between our emotional brain and our thinking brain, and some of the findings are essential in controlling and directing our own actions toward living a rewarding and fulfilling life. The most important of these findings is the fact that our primitive, emotional brain has the ability to totally override our thinking brain.

Whenever we are confronted with situations that we perceive as threatening to our very existence, the quicker-acting emotional brain has a tendency to call all of the shots. It is as if the decision is made that there is no time to think, we must act. In addition, the actions taken tend to deal with basic survival instincts, such as eating.

So even though it may seem irrational to respond to a reduction in our retirement fund by eating cake and ice cream, to our emotional brain it makes perfect sense. While our thinking brain may understand that ingesting an entire pizza with soda will not in any way help clean up the oil spill and save the Gulf of Mexico, our emotional brain compels us to take this age-old solution.

Confusion about how all these modern tragedies could have happened and fear about the future is amplified as the media continue to remind us of how really bad things are. At the same time, our emotional brains are also constantly replaying all the threatening news on a subconscious level. Feeling that our own personal safety is in jeopardy creates deep insecurity. This feeling of insecurity prompts our emotional brain to *"Do something, now!"* Is it any wonder that we feel we are in a constant state of stress and anxiety?

> *As I react to my own story surrounding these current global crises, I'm aware of feeling upset because it seems as though something has been taken away from me without my consent.*
>
> *That "something" is SECURITY.*

Feelings of being out of control can trigger desperate measures to relieve the pain. A tiny voice in my head whispers, "let's eat," and I choose to ignore it. That's my old response to emotional pain that is sneaking up on me, and I am choosing to not answer the call to junk food this time. I know where eating junk food leads me: weight gain, sluggishness, and even more out-of-control feelings. Instead, I make a decision to stop focusing on what is out of my control and make changes in my life that I can indeed control. Gaining weight is not the answer. Staying healthy is.

How are you dealing with the upheavals and challenges in your life? Do you hear a voice whispering or perhaps shouting, "Eat!"

If you, like so many, eat in response to times of uncertainty, stress and tension, remind yourself that food is only a temporary and phony fix with long-term negative consequences. Sugar, fat, and toxic additives will give you an illusion of safety and calm only because of the sedative chemical effects on your brain and nervous system. Eating also acts as a distraction to painful life events. It gives you a false sense of control. Are you ready to stop retreating into a false sense of safety with food? Are you ready to take control of your reactions to challenging life events?

When you talk to yourself with irrational statements of flimsy excuses, victimization and untruths you sabotage your efforts and desires to be healthy and slender. In addition, you make more stress for yourself by gaining weight and feeling disappointed. These irrational statements are the voice of what I call "The Trickster."

Becoming aware of trickster thoughts and how truly disabling they are will allow you to choose another way of viewing life's challenges. When you are in crisis and are about to reach for junk food, ask yourself, *"What thought is seducing me into hurting myself with food?"*

Once you become aware of the irrational thought that is leading you to the irrational response of eating junk food, correct the trickster thought with fact. At first, this takes awareness and effort, similar to learning new phrases in a foreign language. But with time, the trickster thoughts will become less and less intense and you will eventually automatically replace them with rational thoughts. This is the practice of taking control of your thoughts, feelings, and reactions during difficult times. It is a practice that will help bring you closer to a life of freedom from abusing food forever.

Here are some common trickster voices that lead us to eat during times of crisis and examples of how to answer tricks with fact:

- **TRICKSTER THOUGHT:** "I deserve this. Look what I've been through today."

- **FACT:** "I deserve good health, no matter what the events of the day have been."

- **TRICKSTER THOUGHT:** "What the heck. Nothing's going well. I might as well eat."

- **FACT:** "The worst thing I can do is cause more body harm and pain in response to outside chaos. Giving up and giving in are bad choices in times of stress. What I need now is to practice healthy stress management skills."

- **TRICKSTER THOUGHT:** "Everyone's overeating, so I can too."

- **FACT:** "Not everyone is overeating. That's just a trick my mind is playing on me. I am now choosing to disconnect from that reaction (and from that crowd!) and connect with people who are staying healthy. I choose to notice that some people are reacting to stress in positive ways, like working out. Today I choose to hang out with the healthy crowd and when the crisis is over, we'll be physically healthy."

- **TRICKSTER THOUGHT:** "Food is always there for me. I need my comfort food."

- **FACT:** "Lots of things and people are there for me. *I am there for me!* Today I choose to focus on the 'constants' in my life: my family, friends, pets, and hobbies. I refuse to be seduced by the 'comfort food' trick."

The more aware you become of the trickster voice that suggests "let's eat" when crises occur, the better you are able to choose a healthier outcome. You are in control of your thoughts, feelings, and behaviors always. Show the inner trickster the door, and welcome in your inner rational self. There are many healthy ways to deal with crises. Are you willing to practice them?

> *We are what we repeatedly do.*
> *Excellence, then, is not an act, but a habit.*
> —ARISTOTLE

SUCCESS JOURNAL ENTRY

The first step is awareness. Identify the trickster thoughts that emerge when you are in emotional crisis. Next, counteract the trick with fact. Practicing this thought substitution exercise will give you a new and profound sense of personal control.

• *My Trickster Thought:* _____

• *Fact:* _____

• *My Trickster Thought:* _____

• *Fact:* _____

• *My Trickster Thought:* _____

• *Fact:* _____

• *My Trickster Thought:* _____

• *Fact:* _____

• *My Trickster Thought:* _____

• *Fact:* _____

• *My Trickster Thought:* _____

• *Fact:* _____

• *My Trickster Thought:* _____

• *Fact:* _____

Make a commitment to ignore the trickster thoughts, and follow the fact thoughts. After all, don't you deserve to talk to yourself in rational, health-affirming ways?

CHAPTER 16

With each step you take, you will grow stronger and stronger, more and more skilled, more and more self-confident, and more and more successful. —MARK VICTOR HANSEN

Anchoring and Strengthening Your Motivation to Lose Weight

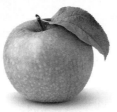

ONE OF THE

BIGGEST CHALLENGES

IN FOLLOWING A WEIGHT loss program is sustaining motivation until you have reached your goal. What starts off with a bang can and does all too often dissipate as time goes on.

However, you can keep your motivation strong and working for you day after day. Just as you select the settings on your washing machine, you can set your motivation levels as well. I have found a technique called "anchoring" to be a very helpful tool in this regard.

> *Anchoring technique:* This is a powerful hypnosis technique that will help you stay powered up and motivated throughout your weight loss program. Use it for instant strength when you feel tempted to eat junk food or when you are thinking of skipping an exercise routine.
>
> It goes like this: Sit or lie down and close your eyes. Try to clear your mind of distracting thoughts and images. Feel yourself relax as you breathe slowly and deeply.
>
> Now mentally drift into your past and go back to a time in your life when you felt very successful and proud of yourself. It can be

any event, such as a personal accomplishment or a particularly happy moment in your life. A memory that elicits the strongest positive emotion works best for this exercise. Patiently wait for this memory to arise. Now imagine reliving the event. Really get into it, as though it's happening right now. Use as many senses as possible to re-experience the event. See it. Hear it. Feel it. Enjoy the happy, secure, proud feelings that arise in your heart as you recall this pleasant time. Let these beautiful feelings grow in intensity. Enjoy the wonderful sensations that are now filling every cell of your body.

Now, when your feelings are really soaring, touch your thumb to your forefinger. As you do so, feel the positive sensations from your memory increase even more. Allow these positive feelings to grow stronger and stronger as you press your thumb and finger together harder. The harder you press, the better you feel. Practice this for as long as you like, and have fun with it. The more intensely you can feel the positive emotions, the stronger the anchor.

This emotional anchor is now yours to use whenever you need a confidence boost. For instance, when you are having difficulty walking away from dessert or are feeling the motivation to exercise beginning to drain away, use your anchor response to remind you of your strength and power. From now on, whenever you wish to feel more confident, just press your thumb and forefinger together, and the good, confident feelings from your pleasant memory will fill you completely.

This anchor is your new tool that can be strengthened at will. When you've stepped on the scale and noticed a weight loss, anchor that great feeling by pressing your thumb and forefinger together. Enjoy the success and anchor it in for future use. After you've completed a workout, anchor that proud feeling as well. Any time you feel proud and happy, build and strengthen your anchoring response. It will be there for you forever.

I was taught this anchoring technique at a hypnosis training seminar over twenty years ago. Although I have since forgotten the specific pleasant memory that I used in the original anchoring exercise, I still get a rush of strength whenever I press my thumb and forefinger together! It's a handy quick tool I use for feeling instant confidence while dealing with challenging situations, such as before public speaking.

■ *ANCHORING STEPS SUMMARY*

1. Get into a relaxed position, close your eyes, and begin to relax your mind and body. Breathe deeply and slowly. Create an intention in your heart and mind of allowing this new technique to work for you.

2. Drift mentally back in time, and recall a time of personal strength, pride, and happiness.

3. Re-live the event with as many senses as possible. Really get into it!

4. Increase the intensity of the emotional recall by pressing your thumb to your forefinger. Allow this movement to anchor the memory.

5. Practice increasing the good feelings by pressing your fingers together while remembering positive feelings and accomplishments from your past.

6. From on now, any time you press your thumb and forefinger together, you will experience an instantaneous wave of happiness and inner strength.

7. Use this technique whenever you wish to feel motivated and confident. For instance, when you feel your motivation to lose weight begin to slacken, just use your emotional anchor and enjoy the boost of inner strength that immediately surges within!

Enjoy!

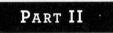

PART II

Developing Your Personal Weight Loss Plan

CHAPTER 17

If we did all the things we are capable of doing,
we would literally astound ourselves.
—THOMAS EDISON

Your Formula for Success

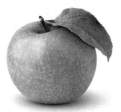

CONGRATULATIONS

ON MAKING GREAT

STRIDES IN RELEASING THE emotional attachment to food! You are now ready to take the next step: adopting a personal eating plan that will allow you to lose weight easily and permanently.

■ *MY STORY*

Several years ago, I visited with a doctor who specializes in endocrinology to discuss my weight issues. I told him that although I had lost twenty-five pounds, my weight loss seemed stuck at a weight that was clearly still unhealthy. He asked me to describe a typical day of eating and exercise. As I recited the foods and portion sizes I commonly ate, I could see him mentally ticking off the calories in his head. He said, "It looks like you're at about 1,700 calories, which is too high for your height and build. I recommend you reduce your daily intake to around 1,200 calories a day." He then personally printed out a lengthy list of foods, their fiber content, and calorie count.

I wondered how I could possibly reduce my caloric intake without feeling even hungrier than I already was. I couldn't imagine eating less than what I was currently eating without feeling famished, weak, and irritable. My discouragement led me to seek the answers.

I started reading any and all books I could get my hands on that gave sound medical advice. I wasn't interested in trendy, outrageous, or potentially harmful diets. I wanted good information about healthy eating. I kept notes of the common denominator ideas that the writers of these books offered and started applying the principles to myself.

Armed with the best weight loss information I could find, I came up with a personal plan that allowed me to shed the pounds without cravings and constant hunger.

■ *A SOUND PLAN TO REDUCE HUNGER, CRAVINGS, AND WEIGHT*

The newest information on weight loss and nutrition suggests that the *type* of calories you eat is just as important to weight loss success as *how many calories you consume.* Taking this into consideration, I found that the most important element to healthy and permanent weight loss is eating whole, good-quality nutritious foods. Foods that are high in nutritional value tend to not only be naturally low in calories, but also make you feel satisfied and energized. I also discovered that when you eat and the pace at which you eat are equally important factors.

I came up with two lists: A "DO" list and a "STAY AWAY FROM" list (which I will share with you later in this chapter). I found that by eating in accordance with the "DO" list, my appetite diminished and my cravings and weight melted away. Many of my clients have had similar success using the plan that I now call *The Formula For Success.*

■ *CALORIES COUNT*

Getting back to the topic of calories, here's what fitness expert Jillian Michaels, in her book *Master Your Metabolism* tells us about calories and weight loss: "Now, before you belly up to the buffet, remember one thing. I've said it a million times, I'll say it again: Calories. Do. Count." *

Although Michaels says that a good weight loss program is not just about calorie counting, it's about health, it's helpful to have an idea of healthy baselines. In her quotes from the American Diabetes Association, Michaels says that if you are an average-sized woman who wants to lose weight, shoot for 1,200 to 1,400 calories a day. A small to moderate-sized man who wants to lose weight should aim to consume 1,600 to 1,900 calories a day. Remember, these are just guidelines. Consult with your doctor to determine the caloric intake that is healthy for you.

■ KEEP A FOOD DIARY

I strongly encourage you to keep a food diary during the beginning stages of your weight loss journey. In addition to writing down what you eat and the calories you consume, also note what you are thinking and feeling when you reach for food, as is illustrated earlier in the book. This serves three purposes.

- First, it will give you the reality check that is so necessary to self-discovery and realistic planning.

- Second, it will keep you in touch with how your thoughts and feelings affect your appetite.

- Third, it will educate you regarding the amount of calories various foods contain. For instance, did you know that just 1 white chunk macadamia cookie contains 250 calories? A chocolate chip muffin has 630 calories! Contrast this to 1 cup of broccoli, which contains 30 calories, and 1 medium egg, which has only 70 calories. And it's not just the calories, but also the cravings that get set up when you indulge in sugary, greasy foods. I don't know anyone who gets overwhelming cravings for broccoli or eggs, but plenty of people are addicted to ice cream, chips, and cookies.

When I began my food diary, I used a handy food calorie paper-back book, which I tucked in my purse for easy reference. There are several excellent websites and applications that will provide you with the calorie count of foods as well. Some of my clients conveniently use their electronic devices to note their daily consumption. Some just carry a small notepad. Do whatever it takes to make your food diary easy to use. For your convenience, I have included a food diary journal page at the end of this chapter.

■ *THE FORMULA FOR SUCCESS*

With my plan called the "Formula," there are delicious, nutritious foods you eat on a daily basis. And most importantly, you do eat! Never starve yourself. With the "Formula" you will have energy to burn and your weight can just melt away.

■ *BEGINNING THE "FORMULA"*

First, consider beginning with a medically approved food elimination diet to determine any food sensitivities. An elimination diet can help you discover which food items are not beneficial to you and if you should restrict those items in your diet.

I personally used Dr. Mark Hyman's book, *The UltraSimple Diet*, with excellent success. It was only after doing the elimination diet that I discovered my dairy and gluten sensitivities. Eliminating dairy, gluten, and sugars for two weeks changed me in ways that seemed miraculous at the time. I started to lose weight, lost my cravings, and regulated my hunger. My metabolism kicked into high gear. I had so much energy that I literally had to exercise! It was so wonderful that I decided to keep the good reaction forever by continuing a nutrition plan that would keep my weight off and my energy level high.

Whether you decide to do an elimination diet is a personal decision. What I can say is that I haven't met anyone yet who has regretted taking that first step. My client, April, had been unable to shed a single pound in years, even though she exercised with a personal trainer several times a week. Deeply discouraged, she came to me for help. When I shared my own success story with her, April decided to try Dr. Hyman's elimination diet for at least a week. April went from discouraged to elated as she lost six pounds her first week! I have had numerous clients and friends who have enjoyed similar success stories.

After doing a healthy food elimination diet, if desired (and if approved by your doctor), you can use these simple guidelines that my clients and I have followed for losing weight and maintaining the weight loss. Adjust them to fit your specific medical needs, tastes, and food sensitivities.

HERE IS THE "FORMULA":

- Eat breakfast every day.
- Eat healthy sources of protein with every meal.
- Eat unlimited amounts of vegetables daily (buy organic whenever possible).
- Eat whole grains (if you are not gluten sensitive).
- Eat every three to four hours. (Eat slowly, chewing your food thoroughly.)
- Stop eating three hours before bedtime.
- Eat fruit separately from a meal, as a snack.
- Drink lots of water and herbal tea daily.
- Use healthy oils, such as olive, flaxseed, and coconut oil.
- Snack on small portions of unsalted nuts (if not allergic) and seeds.
- Substitute almond milk if you have dairy sensitivities.

STAY AWAY FROM:

- Refined sugar in all forms.
- Noncaloric sweeteners.
- All sodas, especially diet sodas.
- Fried foods.
- Processed foods that contain artificial flavorings and additives.
- White flour products (bread, pasta, crackers) and white rice.
- High fat dairy products, like whole cheese, and whole milk.
- Alcohol, except sparingly. (Sip that occasional glass of wine slowly.)

That's it in a nutshell! When you find a plan that gives you the body of your dreams and the health you deserve, no matter what your age, it's easy to stay away from foods and behaviors that hurt you. Everything you put into your mouth affects your mood and your biology. It's up to you to decide how to live and what to eat.

The next chapters will help you follow the "Formula" with ease and success. Read on!

Use this chart to graph your progress and program your subconscious mind to support you.

DAILY FOOD JOURNAL

Date	Time	What I Ate (Include Portions)	Calories	How I Was Feeling

At the end of each day, review your journal and note your patterns relating to when you eat, and how your feelings may affect what and how much you eat.

* Michaels, Jillian, *Master Your Metabolism*, (Crown Publishing, 2009), p 87.

CHAPTER 18

Great things are not done by impulse,
but by a series of small things brought together.
—VINCENT VAN GOGH

The No Failure Plan

BECAUSE THIS IS

STRICTLY NOT A DIET,

I ENCOURAGE YOU TO let go the old all-or-nothing diet mentality. The all-or-nothing mentality is about perfection and failure. Within this mindset, when you waver from your diet, even with one snack or meal, your inner critic voice says, "I screwed up, it's over. I might as well go back to my old ways of eating."

Because most traditional diets make us feel deprived, hungry, and irritable, going back to eating sweets and fried foods can be very tempting when we are hard on ourselves! However, giving in to this inner scolding only creates a sense of guilt and failure, which can sadly lead us to overeat once again. This is how the cycle of diet-failure-overeat-diet-failure-overeat begins and continues.

In an August 2010 *Psychology Today Magazine* article, "The New Quitter," the author observes:

> *The abstinence-only doctrines that once dominated the thinking about addiction have given way to a more flexible and more forgiving approach. The trick is to view an episode of backsliding as a chance to learn, an opportunity to develop better techniques for anticipating and avoiding or overcoming urges.*

■ *STOP THE YO-YO CYCLE*

First, let's get rid of the failure words in your mental conversation:

- *Screwed up*
- *Mistake*
- *Messed up*
- *It's over*
- *I'm a failure*

Instead, view a relapse as an opportunity to learn new coping skills and to keep your focus positive. See yourself as a strong, determined person who will lose the weight and keep it off forever. When you use the tools discussed in this book, such as positive self-talk, visualization, and hypnosis, your weight loss journey can be remarkably easy and fun.

■ *THERE ARE NO FAILURES, ONLY LESSONS*

Many people experience relapses on their journey to final success. If you have a minor relapse, ask yourself, "What events or emotions precipitated my overeating?" Make a plan to handle that situation differently next time, and visualize executing the plan in your mind. In this way, you never give up hope but are always learning more about yourself. With knowledge and self-compassion, you will become stronger and more determined to reach your weight loss goal.

I often tell my weight loss clients:

It's not what you do now and then that hurts you, but what you do every day. You are overweight partly because your everyday eating is of poor quality, interspersed with spurts of healthy eating. Just switch it around and make your everyday eating clean and nutritious and now-and-then eat something that is not on the good nutrition list.

■ *STRUCTURE AND FLEXIBILITY*

I like to look at a good weight loss plan as resembling a spinal cord. A spinal cord has structure, but it also has flexibility. It bends with your needs. Likewise, your successful weight loss plan has basic, solid rules but it bends with your lifestyle changes and needs. Learn the basic rules and then incorporate them in a personal way into your individual plan. The rules are simply guidelines. Make each rule your own and you will be more likely to follow through.

■ THE BASIC RULES

1. The 90/10 Rule. It's impossible to be 100 percent perfect all of the time, so why set an unrealistic expectation? Instead, aim for following your nutrition plan 90 percent of the week and give yourself permission to eat away from the plan 10 percent of the time. This gives you the emotional space to progress without guilt and shame.

The 90/10 rule was a major shift in my perspective that allowed me to finally lose the weight and keep it off. Use the 90/10 rule in any way that suits your lifestyle and preferences. I like to eat healthy nutritious foods Monday through Friday and enjoy some off-plan food on Saturday or Sunday. A wonderful by-product of eating healthily all week long is that by the weekend, my appetite is smaller and my cravings for junk food are gone. It's a built-in success plan! So, if I decide to eat pie, I now tend to desire a very small portion. It's almost impossible to overindulge.

2. Don't throw in the towel, just make minor adjsutments.
On some days, you're going to be hungrier than on other days. Yesterday, for instance, I felt physically hungry all day. This was not "head hunger," but real my-body-needs-fuel-hunger. So I gave myself permission to eat more. I simply ate more of the foods that physically nourish me and stayed away from junk food, breads, and sugar. Today, to balance it out, I will eat less food than on a normal day, but I know this will be easy because the hunger has now subsided.

It's perfectly fine that I ate more calories than usual yesterday, because I will make the adjustment today by having fewer calories. As long as I eat foods that nourish me and avoid eating starchy, greasy, sugary foods, my weight stays balanced even when I eat more during one or two days of the week. It's all about listening to your body and making conscious, healthy decisions to feed your body nourishing food.

I recommend to my clients to not focus just on the day at hand, but to look at the whole week. In this way, they won't throw in the towel when they have one bad day.

"Counteract the overeating on Sunday by eating a couple hundred calories less on Monday," I say to them. "Just don't overreact and quit your program." This not only builds in some flexibility, but also allows us to learn how to stay consistently focused on the long-term goal.

3. The Three-Bites Rule. If you really feel like indulging in dessert, enjoy three or four bites and then leave or share the rest. A few bites eaten slowly and with joy are much more satisfying than a whole pie quickly and guiltily wolfed down. Remember, you are working on ending the guilt/overeating cycle, so if you choose to eat sweets, choose to do so with happiness.

An average sized restaurant dessert typically contains three hundred to six hundred calories; so eating just a few bites keeps your calorie intake to around one hundred calories.

4. Say "no" to second helpings. Keep your meal in the pots and pans on the stove or countertop, not on the table in front of you. That way, if you are tempted to grab a second helping, you have to first get up and walk to the stove. Better yet, make it a rule to take a few minutes break before helping yourself to seconds.

Break the overeating trance state you can get into during a meal by distracting yourself before reaching for seconds. How you distract yourself is up to you. Perhaps walk around a bit, open the mail, get some water. Then, if you're still hungry, have a small second helping. Chances are, however, that you won't be hungry and will be able to get on with the day feeling satisfied, not overly full.

5. Take a stroll after eating dinner. Ideally, take a fifteen-minute stroll after your evening meal to burn up the sugar (remember, even vegetables have sugar) and to keep your body in fat burning mode while you sleep. The worst thing to do is to lie on the couch after dinner watching TV or napping. Resting after dinner only puts your body into a fat storage mode.*

6. **Finish eating three hours before going to bed.** A nutritionist once told me that digesting food is considered work by the digestive track. Therefore, eating right before bed is forcing your body to work overtime, like a factory that never gets to shut down. Because your body is tired at night, it turns the food you just ate into fat instead of burning it as fuel. Doesn't it make sense, then, to act compassionately toward your body, especially your digestive tract, by letting it shut down while you sleep? Your body can handle the job of digesting food better in the morning, and you'll experience a deeper night of sleep as well.

7. **Move your body every day.** My clients often ask me, "When's the best time of day to exercise?" My answer is, "Whenever you'll do it!" The basic rule is to move your body every day, but how and when you do that is entirely up to you. Remember that the benefits of movement are cumulative during the course of the day, so you may want to do a quick workout in the morning and then take a walk after dinner. Or, if it fits your schedule, do a cardio workout after work. Stay flexible and realistic. Not many of us can commit to a whole hour of exercise at the gym seven days a week, 365 days of the year, but we can commit to moving our bodies as much as possible throughout the day.

For example, I've found that my brain works best right after rising. So, on the days that I will be doing a lot of cognitive work, such as writing a chapter of this book, I'll put off my morning exercise until later in the day. I've found that daily exercise makes me feel better and because I deserve to feel good, it makes sense to me to make some form of exercise a daily habit. Some days, I do the elliptical for forty-five minutes, and other days I do only fifteen minutes. Some days I walk around the neighborhood lake one time; other days I circle the lake twice.

Some days I choose to bike or to enjoy the thirty-minute resistance circuit at Curves. And there are some days, for whatever reason, I don't exercise at all. Instead of getting down on myself, I calmly make the decision to do a little more exercise the following day.

Some people assume that because I exercise almost daily, that I must love it. The truth is, on some days, I don't even like it! But I *love* the results and that's what I keep my eye on. Exercise, even a small amount each day, is congruent with my long-term goal of being slender, fit, and healthy. The svelte Dr. Oz, of *The Dr. Oz Show*, begins each day with a seven-minute mat workout. This, and his habit of walking quickly and taking stairs instead of elevators, is his daily discipline. When he can, he adds in yoga, short runs, and basketball games with friends (Dr. Do-It-All, *New York Times Magazine*, 2010).

I happen to like variety in my schedule. While I prefer to exercise first thing in the morning, I don't emotionally beat myself up if I decide to do something else (like sleep in!) instead. But I do set the intention to exercise at least twenty minutes that day before I go to bed. As with eating, don't just look at today, but view your goals in terms of the whole week and you'll be more likely to succeed. And remember, try to find some form of exercise that is fun for you and keep in mind that "a little bit goes a long way!"

To further motivate you, I asked an expert in the fitness arena some key questions about exercise and weight loss. My friend, Elizabeth Bowden, is a nutritional consultant and Curves coach who I've watched inspire countless women during my eight years exercising at Curves for Women. Here are my questions and her answers:

- **What advice do you have for overweight people about getting and staying motivated to exercise?**

  Find what works for you and your body in the moment. Beginning anything new takes time, and learning to use your body to achieve its best results takes patience. Do not feel you have to force yourself to a routine. Find as many ways as you can to make movement count as exercise throughout the day.

- **Why is it so important to exercise for heath and well-being?**

  When we exercise, the body releases hormones and chemicals that literally enhance our well-being. That can be a powerful thing to tap into. Overcoming a challenge can make us feel good about ourselves, and setting reasonable, attainable goals about exercise can be quite rewarding.

• **What is the best way to burn calories and fat with the least amount of time and effort?**

Calories from food are the energy the body uses for everything it does. Remember, "energy in" affects "energy out" and vice versa. The best way to burn calories and fat is to keep eating! The body needs a lot of energy to break down stored fats. If you do not eat healthy and natural foods while trying to lose weight, it's harder for the body to find balance. In order for the body to release stored fat, you must consume healthy fat (such as Omega 3).

• **What are the main qualities you see in people who are the most successful at sticking with their exercise plan?**

People who realize that their health is in their hands are the most successful. Many times the only control we have in our lives at the moment is what we put into our mouths and how much we move our bodies. When someone is willing to acknowledge the challenge of losing weight and focuses on maintaining a healthy body, they will succeed.

* Rosedale, Ron, M.D., *The Rosedale Diet*, (Collins Living, 2005), p 183.

CHAPTER 19

Stand up to your obstacles and do something about them.
You will find that they haven't half the strength you think they have.
—NORMAN VINCENT PEALE

Identify and Neutralize Your Triggers

PEOPLE, EVENTS,

EMOTIONS, AND FOODS

THAT ACT AS PERSONAL conditioned stimuli to overeating are called triggers. These are the situations that make it difficult to ignore the inner voice that says, "What the heck. Let's eat!" By causing us to feel momentarily uninhibited, unmotivated, and undisciplined, they can easily sabotage a weight loss program. In the midst of these stimuli, it's as though a window opens and all of our good weight loss intentions fly out!

Your overeating reactions in the presence of these stimuli are unconsciously conditioned and have nothing to do with willpower or self-discipline. In fact, I strongly believe that situational triggers actually induce automatic hypnotic states that cause us to temporarily lose control of our appetite and food choices. In the midst of an overeating trance, we are unaware of how much or what we're eating. We lose track of time and stop caring about the calories we're consuming. We lose control.

Are there people, events, or places in your life that make it seemingly impossible to stick to your weight loss plan? If so, it's time to acknowledge your unique triggers and to build a strong strategy plan.

And no, your strategy plan does not require extreme action. You do not need to divorce your spouse, quit your job, or move to a deserted part of the world that is devoid of restaurants! It simply requires a change in mindset that will neutralize the sabotaging power of your triggers.

Take a few moments to complete the following inventory. I have included a sample inventory and strategy plan as a guide. Your completed strategy plan will allow you to take control of the triggers that may have been bossing your cravings and appetite around and to stay focused on your weight loss plan.

■ *MY PERSONAL TRIGGERS INVENTORY:*

1. *With whom do I overeat or eat unhealthy foods?*

2. *Which social settings cause me to eat in unhealthy ways?*

3. *Which foods trigger cravings?*

4. *Which emotions cause me to reach for junk food or to overeat?*

5. *What time of day do I experience cravings that I have a hard time saying no to?*

6. *Other triggers for me:*

My strategy plan to counteract my triggers:

1. _____

2. _____

3. _____

4. _____

5. _____

6. _____

■ *SAMPLE PERSONAL TRIGGERS INVENTORY:*

1. *With whom do I overeat or eat unhealthy foods?*

- My spouse
- My best friend

2. *Which social settings cause me to eat in unhealthy ways?*
- Friday night Happy Hour with my work colleagues
- All restaurants

3. *Which foods trigger cravings?*

- Potato chips
- Chocolate chip cookies
- Candy, especially red licorice

4. *What emotions cause me to reach for junk food or to overeat?*

- Anger, boredom

5. *What time of day do I experience cravings that I have a hard time saying no to?*
- 3:00 in the afternoon
- Evenings, between 7:00 and 10:00

6. *Other triggers for me:*

- Driving by fast food restaurants

■ *SAMPLE STRATEGY PLAN TO COUNTERACT TRIGGERS:*

1. I will remind myself that my spouse and best friend have the right to eat as they wish. I will tell them that I am committed to losing weight, but have no expectation or need for them to change their eating patterns. The only person who needs to change is me. I will imagine my spouse and best friend feeling comfortable in my presence as I eat in a healthy manner and lose weight.

2. As I drive to Happy Hour or restaurants, I will imagine myself thoroughly enjoying the company of friends without overeating and eating junk food. I will tell myself, "*Socializing is more about talking than eating. I have more fun when I'm eating small portions of healthy food and feeling in control.*"

3. I am surrounding myself with healthy alternatives at home and at work. I will mentally see myself calmly and proudly walking away from junk food.

4. I am making a list of ways to deal with anger and boredom without eating. I will review and follow this list until the new responses become automatic.

5. I recognize that mid-afternoon cravings are more about feeling tired, than about being hungry. I will close my eyes for a few minutes of rest at 3 pm. If I feel physically hungry after my rest, I will enjoy a small snack of fruit and a cup of herbal tea.

I will now say to myself: *"The desire to eat in the evening is an old, conditioned response that I can alter. I will now enjoy reading and watching TV without eating. The kitchen is off limits to me after dinner."* I will visualize this happening.

6. As I drive by fast food restaurants, I will smell the grease and remember how fat, starch, and sugars, cause me to gain weight and to feel tired. I now imagine driving by the fast food restaurants with a smile on my face as I go home to prepare a healthy meal. I imagine the money I used to spend on fast food building in my bank account. I will enjoy this extra money by getting a massage once a month.

You now have a powerful strategy plan that will neutralize your triggers. Enjoy the feelings of control and confidence as you continue to lose weight no matter who or what show up in your daily life!

CHAPTER 20

*You have a very powerful mind that can make
anything happen as long as you keep yourself centered.*

—WAYNE DYER

Eating Mindfully

Eat Until You're Satisfied, Not Until You're Full

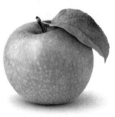

FOR PERMANENT

WEIGHT LOSS, ONE OF

THE MOST IMPORTANT POINTS to keep in mind is to never eat until you feel full. I know that this is completely counterintuitive, as it's most likely a built-in evolutionary mechanism.

When food was much less available, people feasted and fattened up to store energy in order to stay alive during times of famine. The feast and famine way of eating was a survival instinct, and those who could eat the most when food was plentiful survived to have offspring. However, today food is in abundance all year round, and we seem to have gotten into the feast mode of eating nonstop.

The holiday feasting is happening almost daily now, with huge meals eaten in the many restaurants that are in all cities. In addition, people commonly binge on weekends, justifying their choice by referencing a stressful workweek or feeling too exhausted to care about health and weight loss.

Most Americans eat until they're at full or over-full capacity. We like that full belly feeling. But isn't it true that within ten to fifteen minutes, you're feeling overly stuffed and sluggish? Are you searching for the couch or bed to collapse into?

The way thin people eat is that they eat small portions and stop before they're full. For appetite control, tell yourself, *"I eat until I'm gently satisfied."* That way, the word "satisfied" gives you a pleasant feeling and keeps you from feeling deprived. The word "gently" reminds you to be gentle with your body. The stomach is a very sensitive organ that is literally lined with a dense network of nerves. These nerves cause you to feel butterflies when you are nervous and nauseated when you are upset. It is a feeling organ. It deserves your respect.

Studies have shown that using a smaller plate will trick your mind into thinking that you've eaten more. In these studies, people given bigger portions eat what they're served. Other studies have shown that people given bigger plates at a buffet eat more calories than people given smaller plates.*

The Japanese have the term: "hara hachi bunme," which refers to eating until their stomach is only 2/3 full. Many people believe that it's this practice of stopping eating before they are completely full that keep the Japanese people not only thin, but some of the longest living people on Earth.

■ *PRESENT MOMENT EATING EXERCISE:*

By eating slowly and consciously, smaller portions are more filling. This practice is called "mindfulness."

To help my workshop participants connect with the joy of truly savoring food, I often facilitate this mindfulness exercise. I encourage you to try it yourself.

1. Select a tasty healthy food, preferably one that has a chewy consistency. I often use nuts or pieces of dried fruit in my workshops.

2. Place one piece of the food in your hand and look at it. Imagine where it was grown, who cared for it, and how it came into your life. Look at its color, shape, and texture.

3. Smell the food and enjoy its aroma. What does it smell like? What childhood memories, perhaps, does it elicit?

4. Now place this bite of food into your mouth and begin to chew it slowly. What is the immediate flavor as you first bite into it? How does its taste change as you continue to chew? What is its texture? Chew slowly and enjoy the taste of this morsel of food. You've begun the digestion process of this food and so connect with how the nutrients are already beginning to enter your bloodstream. You are already feeling healthier and better by chewing this tasty bite. Savor every bite. Enjoy slowly chewing this delicious food.

5. Only after thoroughly chewing the food, swallow it. Imagine it entering your stomach for further digestion. Your mind is registering that food has entered your stomach. Feel your stomach accepting this bite of food and beginning to digest it further.

The most common reaction I get from my workshop participants is that they were enjoying chewing their morsel so completely that they didn't want to swallow it and end the enjoyment! Isn't this the opposite of how we usually eat? Observe people eating, especially if they're in a hurry, and notice that they barely chew their food. Instead, they gulp it down.

I was observing a young man at the airport one day. His girlfriend brought him a huge Mexican take-out meal in a Styrofoam box. He opened the container, took the plastic fork, and started shoveling the food in massive forkfuls into his mouth. He barely chewed once or twice before gulping it down. I watched with amazement how quickly and mindlessly he consumed at least 2,000 calories and didn't even seem to enjoy it. What's more, his brain didn't have time to register that all of those calories had been eaten. My guess is that he was quite hungry an hour or so later, looking for another starchy meal or snack.

If he had slowed down and chewed more intentionally, it is reasonable to surmise that he would have been full before finishing his meal. His brain would have gotten the signal "enough" half way through the meal, and he would have lost interest in it. Throwing food away when you're full and when you're not in a position to keep leftovers (like at the airport) is better than treating your stomach like a garbage can. Whenever you eat beyond stomach fullness, it is waste and turns into ugly fat. Better to throw it into a real garbage receptacle than push it down into your stomach and overfill your fat cells.

Start being an observer of how people (including you) eat.

Notice if they're enjoying the process of eating or just gulping food. Begin to notice how you eat when you're alone. Are you a shoveler or a food connoisseur?

Like millions of others these days, I enjoy watching the cooking channels on TV. I particularly enjoy observing the judges automatically use the mindfulness way of eating. They first look at the food and comment on the colors and the presentation. They then take a small amount on their fork and often bring it to their nose to smell it. They slowly put the bite of food into their mouth and begin to chew it many times. After slowly chewing, savoring, and swallowing a few bites, they comment on the quality of the food, how they enjoyed the texture and taste, and how the taste changed as they chewed. They often mention how the flavor lingered on their tongue after swallowing.

When you're dining, imagine you're a professional food critic. Notice what you're eating and whether it's pleasing to you. Eat slowly and mindfully, and I guarantee that you will not only enjoy your meal more but you will eat much less than if you had mindlessly gulped it down.

The *Prevention* Magazine article, "Chew More, Eat Less" (October 2009) cited a study in the *American Journal of Clinical Nutrition* that demonstrates the significance of chewing and weight loss. The study showed that people who chewed almonds twenty-five to forty times felt fuller and more satisfied than when they only chewed ten times. The researchers also found that the "steady chewers" absorbed more healthy unsaturated fats and broke down more fiber, releasing more nutrients into their bloodstream.

Intrigued with these results, I decided to do the experiment with myself. I cooked a breakfast of eggs and black beans two mornings in a row. Each breakfast had the same quantity of food. On the first morning, I ate the breakfast at a relatively fast pace, while reading a magazine. I was finished in just a few minutes and was left wanting more food. I just didn't feel satisfied.

The next morning, I ate mindfully. The magazine was gone. Just me and the plate of food on the table. I looked at the food I had prepared and actually noticed how good it looked. I could smell the spiciness of the salsa seasoning the beans. I ate each bite slowly, really tasting the food and its flavor. I spent a good fifteen minutes thoroughly enjoying the breakfast and felt satisfied and calm after eating.

After both meals, I went to my office to see clients. The effects of the two different eating paces became evident while I worked. The first morning, I felt famished within ninety minutes of eating breakfast. Although I had eaten plenty of good, nourishing protein and fiber, I was very hungry. After the second morning, however, I felt strong and satiated for over three hours before beginning to feel hungry again.

I've encouraged my clients to try this experiment, and every one of them had the same results. Food eaten quickly and without enjoyment just didn't seem to "stick" with them, and they were hungering for more food immediately after eating or soon afterward. When they ate slowly, however, they sometimes couldn't even finish their meal. They were too full and this fullness lasted for several hours. Because they ultimately consumed fewer calories with this way of eating, they couldn't help but lose weight. In this way, they were not feeling deprived or hungry while losing weight.

My sister Janice and I like to take a spring trip to Mexico every year and have found a favorite all-inclusive resort with excellent cooking. To thoroughly enjoy the cuisine without gaining even one pound of weight, we use the mindfulness way of eating. We carefully plan what foods we'll enjoy: the fresh fruits and vegetables, the delicious seafood, omelets, and fresh juice. We are intentional about how we feed our bodies. We look at the huge table filled with cakes, cookies, and other sugary delicacies, without a strong urge to indulge in them. We just enjoy how beautiful they look and marvel at the pastry chef's artistry and skill. This doesn't mean we never eat any of the desserts. After all, we are on vacation. But we carefully choose some special delicacies and share them. We savor them slowly and feel very satisfied with just a small amount of sweets.

How do we resist bingeing on the sugar? We both know, from past experience, the consequences of that behavior. It would cause a crash in energy within an hour or two and give us sugar cravings the rest of the vacation. Eating large amounts of refined sugar and white flour products would have us packing annoying cravings and extra body fat along with our luggage on our trip home! Why bother? It takes just a minute to hurriedly eat hundreds of calories and fat in desserts, but a lot longer to lose the consequent weight gain.

If you're vacationing, enjoy small amounts of desserts and then push away from the table. Focus on the fun things you can enjoy that have nothing to do with eating, such as swimming, napping on the beach, walking, playing, and reading.

■ *CONDUCTING YOUR OWN MINDFULNESS EXPERIMENT:*

Eat a meal (can be breakfast, lunch, or dinner) at a fast pace, preferably while watching TV or reading.

After the meal, ask yourself these questions: Use a 1 to 10 scale.

1. How enjoyable was the eating experience?
2. How satisfied do I feel, in terms of hunger?
3. How does my stomach feel?

Stay tuned to your hunger cues, and note how long after your meal you begin to feel hungry or to crave a snack. How is your energy level? Does it stay even?

Now, repeat this experiment the next day. Eat the same meal, but use the mindfulness steps outlined earlier in the chapter. Turn off the TV. Close the book or newspaper. Have nothing present to distract your attention from the meal. Eat slowly, chewing every bite several times, while focusing on the meal and how great it tastes.

Now, evaluate your meal experience.

1. How enjoyable was the eating experience?
2. How satisfied do I feel, in terms of hunger?
3. How does my stomach feel?

Stay tuned to your hunger cues, and note how long after your meal you begin to feel hungry or to crave a snack. How is your energy level? Does it stay even?

Did you notice a difference in results?

Eating intentionally allows you to feel in control of food and of your appetite. Give your stomach the respect and attention it deserves while you savor your meals. Enjoy looking at beautiful desserts like you enjoy looking at artwork. Then enjoy walking away from them with pride and happiness!

SUCCESS JOURNAL ENTRY

Prepare a meal that is colorful, healthy, and inviting.
Enjoy the meal with mindfulness as described above.
Record your experience below:

_____

_____

_____

_____

_____

_____

_____

_____

_____

_____

Research To Practice Series, No. 2, Do Increased Portion Sizes Affect How Much We Eat?, National Center For Chronic Disease Prevention and Health Promotion, Division of Nutrition and Physical Activity.

CHAPTER 21

There is no failure. Only feedback.

—ROBERT ALLEN

Weigh Yourself Regularly

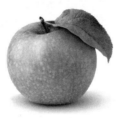

"**I** DON'T NEED TO

WEIGH MYSELF

BECAUSE I JUST GO BY how my clothes are fitting." I hear this statement a lot and was once in that mindset. I owned an old, inaccurate scale that I rarely used. By not weighing myself, I could effectively keep myself in denial as I gained weight.

Another deceptive situation is the stretchable fabric that is used in clothing today. I could gain over ten pounds or more (depending on the fabric) and still fit into my clothes! When I was finally weighed at the doctor's office one day, I was shocked to see how heavy I was. I realized that I had been in massive denial over my weight gain, and stretchy clothes were my allies in denial.

Why weigh yourself regularly? It keeps you in contact with reality and out of denial, which is the only way to seriously lose weight and keep it off.

My client, Ann, never weighed herself until her annual physicals. With every physical for the past five years, she was upset to find out she had gained weight. "I dread going in for my annual," she said. "Its always bad news as I keep getting heavier." In our session, Ann decided to live in reality by facing the truth. And the only way to know the truth is by using a scale.

Although the scale can fluctuate one to three pounds without accurately depicting your true weight, it gives you frequent feedback and a sense of control. After all, it's far easier to lose a few pounds of weight now and then, than to face a weight gain of ten pounds or more at the end of the year.

In fact, Dr. Louis Aronne, in his book *The Skinny On Losing Weight Without Being Hungry*, cites a Cornell University study that compared the weight gain of two groups of freshman women. One group was instructed to weigh themselves only twice—once at the beginning of the semester and lastly at the end of the semester. The other group was instructed to weigh themselves daily. At the end of the semester, the group that only weighed in twice gained an average of six pounds. The women who weighed in daily gained no weight.

Have you ever had the shocking experience of stepping on the scale and seeing that you've gained three pounds overnight? Without knowing why this happens, it's pretty difficult to stay positive when this occurs! Many people react with feelings of guilt, shame, and self-blame, so much so that they are tempted to abandon their diets right then and there.

The truth is that it's normal for your weight to fluctuate daily. However, it's not fat that you are losing and gaining daily, but mostly water and liver weight. The liver can actually store more than five pounds of excess glycogen and water from a day of overeating, whereas it takes 3,500–4,000 extra calories to gain just one pound of body fat. Because it's physically impossible to eat 12,000 extra calories in one day, it's equally impossible to gain three pounds of fat in one day!*

Are you ready to face reality and get into control of your daily weigh-ins? I find it is crucial to use an accurate digital scale every morning. It's your daily dose of reality. Tell yourself, *"I can cope with reality. Staying in illusion only gives me a false sense of security and will keep me stuck in weight gain."*

For those of you who are still thinking that you hate the scale and can't deal with the numbers, let me share what I find helpful in this process.

1. Throw out that old, rusty scale with the red arrow and invest in a good quality digital scale. These are available for between $50 and $150. The old fashioned scales can give you only a vague reading. By getting an accurate reading with a digital scale you'll feel the joy in losing even .25 pounds. You'll also get the truth when you gain even just a little weight. And remember, truth is your best tool for weight loss success.

2. Become firmly convinced that the number you see on the scale does not reflect anything about you as a person. It is only a number reflecting your body weight, including water and glycogen storage in your liver at that moment. Period. The number does not tell you anything about your character, intellect, or worthiness. It does not define you as a person. There is no reason whatsoever to feel shame or guilt when you see the number on your scale.

3. View your scale as a friend that is giving you valuable, life-saving information. Love, respect, and honor yourself for having the courage to seek the truth.

4. Over time, it gets easier to step on the scale and look at the results. As you begin to lose weight, you'll actually look forward to weighing in! What was once scary can soon become uplifting.

5. Remember that it's normal to have one to three pounds fluctuation daily, especially as the day goes on. This is due to temporary body waste, food, and water. One of my clients noticed that even drinking a glass of water caused a one-pound increase on the scale! To minimize the fluctuation as much as possible, weigh yourself at the same time every morning, ideally before eating or drinking. This will give you the most accurate reading for the day.

When you're first starting your weight loss program, get an accurate measurement of your weight on Day 1. Then follow your new eating and exercise habits for a week. This will give your body time to get the metabolism kicked up and give you an opportunity to see results the next time you step on the scale. Weigh yourself weekly until you feel ready to weigh-in every morning. I logged my weight every Tuesday morning while I was in my active weight loss program. When I got within twenty pounds of my goal, I started to weigh myself every few days and then moved to daily weighing. Now I continue to weigh myself daily just to keep in touch with my body and eating habits.

This is your weight loss program, and only you can decide the best weigh-in schedule for you. You may decide to weigh yourself every morning, beginning immediately, or to do weekly weigh-ins for a while. The important thing is to use your scale on a regular basis and stay objective and knowledgeable when viewing the numbers. Expect to have a higher number the day after holiday feasting. Then, set a firm expectation to return to a healthy eating and exercise pattern right away.

I now view my scale as a valuable reality check tool. I used to dread stepping on the scale, and now I enjoy it, even if it tells me I've gained a few pounds. It's far easier to deal with a few extra pounds than with the shock of finding out I've gained ten, twenty, or thirty pounds! At this point, I can't imagine a healthy life without my scale.

*Aronne, Louis, M.D., *The Skinny on Losing Weight without Being Hungry*, (Doubleday, 2009), pp. 157, 162.

SUCCESS JOURNAL ENTRY

Commitment to Myself

TODAY, I agree to purchase a digital scale and I further commit to weigh myself regularly and to keep a journal record of my weight.

Signed this _____ *day of* _____ ,

20_____

_____
Signature

■ *SUCCESS JOURNAL ENTRY—MY WEIGHT LOG*

Decide to weigh yourself at least every week, with more frequent weigh-ins as you lose weight. Weigh yourself first thing in the morning, after using the bathroom, and jot the number in your journal. If you find yourself becoming too emotionally attached to the numbers you see, pretend you are an experimenter objectively noting the results of a research study.

Although you will have slight fluctuations daily, you should see a definite downward trend over the course of one or two weeks. My client, Becky, decided to weigh herself daily, right at the beginning of her weight loss program. She discovered that her weight stayed the same from Monday to Friday and then dropped significantly every Saturday. Becky said that if she hadn't kept going, all the way to the weekend, with her weigh-ins, she would have given up that first Friday and gone back to her old eating habits. The old familiar thought of "See, nothing works for me!" would have caused her to quit her program too early, she told me. At the time of this writing, Becky has lost forty-nine pounds and plans to lose another twenty. She weighs herself daily and loves the results!

Becky's discovery is a wonderful reminder that each body reacts differently to the same diet plan. The key is to learn how your body responds to the eating and exercise changes you are making and to keep going, day by day. Many of my clients have the same weight reading for two weeks and then suddenly see a big plunge. It's crucial to know your body's pattern of weight loss by regularly using your scale and keeping a journal. This way, you won't panic or give up when you experience a plateau. Just keep going and know the weight will melt off at the pace that is perfect for your body.

Keeping this weight record not only shows you that you are making positive changes, but just like your food diary, you are programming your subconscious mind daily with your goal. Trust that keeping this journal and your food diary is one of the most powerful strategies you can employ to reach your goals joyfully, steadily, and permanently.

I still keep my success journal and like to glance at it during a low-confidence day. It gives me an instant jolt of pride when I see what I accomplished. I suggest you do the same!

MY WEIGHT LOSS SUCCESS CHART

Starting Weight and Measurements: _____

Goal Weight: _____

Date	Daily Weight Record	Time of Day Weighed

CHAPTER 22

Life is like an ever-shifting kaleidoscope—
a slight change, and all patterns alter.

—SHARON SALZBERG

Seven Secret Weapons
to Keeping Hunger Away

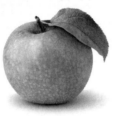

IT DOESN'T

TAKE MUCH TO

MASTER YOUR APPETITE. These seven rules will help you control your cravings:

1. **Eat fiber-rich vegetables and nuts.** Fiber burns slowly, allowing you to feel satisfied longer. Fiber also reduces your appetite by keeping your blood sugar levels at an even keel.*

Tip: I always keep a small bag of unsalted, raw almonds with me to snack on throughout the day, which keeps my appetite manageable and eliminates cravings for bread and sugar.

2. **Eat early.** I try to eat most of my daily calories before dinnertime, and I never skip breakfast. When I fill up with high fiber, high nutrition foods early in the day, I avoid the late afternoon and evening hunger and cravings. Eating early is a definite appetite suppressor, causing me to want only a light dinner and to have very little need or desire for evening snacking. The last thing my body needs after a long day of work is huge quantities of food to digest! Remember, digesting food takes energy and your body has more energy early in the day. Give your body a break when it's tired by keeping food intake to a minimum at night.

3. Eat often. In the *New York Times Magazine* article, "Dr. Do-It-All" (April 12, 2010), author Frank Bruni shares a behind-the-scenes look into the production of the popular medical advice TV show, *The Dr. Oz Show*.

The star of the show, Dr. Mehmut Oz, sometimes referred to as "America's Doctor," is a prominent cardiothoracic surgeon who works at a near-feverish pace from 7 am to 6 pm most days. Using the show to "exhort Americans to tend to all aspects of their health, from head to toe, before they reach a point of no return," Dr. Oz practices what he preaches about how to maintain a healthy body.

At the time of the article, Dr. Oz was 49-years-old, 6 feet tall and weighed 178 pounds. According to Bruni, who spent considerable time with Oz while writing the article:

I never saw him without a portable larder of baggies, plastic containers and thermoses of food and drink, and all of it—every crumb, every drop— was healthful. Roughly every 45 to 60 minutes, as if on cue, he would ingest something from his movable buffet, but only a little bit, his portions assiduously regulated, like an intravenous drip of nutrition. Oz's energy is astounding, intimidating, ludicrous.

I mention Dr. Oz's story as demonstration that we can have a very stressful, insanely busy life and still eat healthily and stay fit. Although you may not want to or need to eat in as structured a manner as Dr. Oz, take note that it is possible to eat frequently, in small amounts, throughout the day. It takes making your health a priority and taking the time to plan ahead. I also travel and navigate my everyday life with my own portable buffet of healthy food. I feel better and more energetic when I eat five mini-meals of nutritious foods. Keeping my blood sugar levels at an even keel, my appetite stays under control and I stay at a healthy weight without counting calories.

4. Start your day with healthy forms of protein. The Greek etymology of the word "protein" is "of first importance." Start your day with some protein, and you'll be nourishing your muscles, organs, skin, teeth, bones, blood, nails, and hair.

Some good sources of protein are eggs, nuts and nut butters, legumes, seeds, lean meat, poultry, yogurt, good quality protein shakes and bars, leafy green vegetables (especially spinach and kale), brown rice, seafood, brussels sprouts, broccoli, soy products, cauliflower, veggie burgers, and hummus. Keep in mind that plant protein has less fat and more fiber than animal protein.

Choose from the list, depending on your preferences and body needs. For instance, I choose to not eat dairy products, but I do eat other animal protein. Again, get to know your body and what foods make your body feel healthy, energized, slender, and fit.

5. Eat protein with every meal. Protein cuts down on hunger, burns slowly, and keeps your carbohydrate cravings to a minimum throughout the day. If you feel you absolutely must have some carbohydrates for breakfast, like cereal, bagels, or toast, accompany it with protein.

A great power breakfast is eggs (poached, soft boiled, or hard boiled), turkey sausage, or beans. The more filling beans are the darker ones, like black or red kidney beans. Lighter colored beans, such as cannellini and pinto beans, have less fiber and can cause an upsurge in blood sugar levels and hunger.

6. Keep moving! Many of my clients learn to respond to artificial "head hunger," as opposed to "stomach hunger," by doing a brief exercise stint. They are astonished to find that after just a few minutes of moving, their appetite is diminished and the hunger goes away. In fact, doing some light exercise after dinner can greatly diminish your need to snack before bedtime. My client, Edward, discovered that while in the past he would automatically reach for some sugary, salty, or starchy carbohydrate snack as soon as he felt hungry in the evening he now goes for a ten-minute walk with his dog. With this plan, he has been able to stop the evening snacking ritual and has lost eight pounds. His dog is happier and healthier as well!

7. Drink water. Years ago, when a friend whom I hadn't seen in a year or so visited I noticed she had lost considerable weight. "How did you lose the weight?" I asked. She replied, "Simple. I read that we often confuse thirst with hunger, so whenever I think I want to eat,

I drink a glass of water instead!" I also have found that drinking water throughout the day diminishes hunger, keeps my skin hydrated and soft, and gives me a wonderful energy boost.

Upon awakening in the morning, remember to drink eight ounces of water right away to rehydrate after several hours of sleeping. Continue to drink water throughout the day and notice how much more energetic you feel. As much as possible, minimize your intake of caffeinated beverages, like soda and coffee. They are very dehydrating. Likewise, limit your intake of fruit juices, which are high in sugar.

Hyman, Mark, M.D., *UltraMetabolism*, (Atria Books, 2007), p. 93.

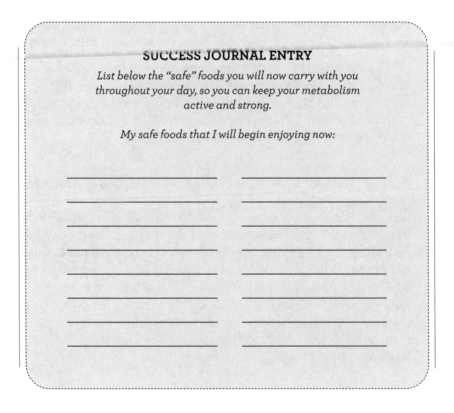

SUCCESS JOURNAL ENTRY
List below the "safe" foods you will now carry with you throughout your day, so you can keep your metabolism active and strong.

My safe foods that I will begin enjoying now:

CHAPTER 23

One cannot think well, love well, sleep well, if one has not dined well.

—VIRGINIA WOOLF

Taking the "Formula" Out to Dinner

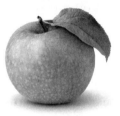

MANY OF MY

CLIENTS, ESPECIALLY

THOSE WHO TRAVEL FREQUENTLY, complain that eating healthily is difficult at restaurants. Heartbreakingly, their lost pounds are quickly gained during vacation or on a business trip. Because I enjoy both travel and healthy weight, I have found ways of dining at restaurants that are conducive to weight loss and maintenance. In fact, I often lose weight when I travel! So can you.

Here are some simple rules for eating out. Remember, all new rules become habit with practice.

- Patronize restaurants that will customize your meals in accordance with your nutritional needs. In other words, spend your money wisely. Spending a few extra dollars for a nutritious meal will save you money in health care costs in the long run. Pretend that fast food restaurants do not exist! After awhile, you'll cease to notice them.

- Tell the waitperson "No bread or chip basket, please." Why tempt yourself unnecessarily? Ask for hot or cold water or tea before ordering your meal.

- Let your eyes wander immediately to the fish, poultry, or salad section of the menu. Ignore the red meat and pasta entrees. An excellent entrée choice is fish or chicken with steamed veggies or salad. Most restaurants offer grilled chicken or seafood on a bed of greens.

- If your entrée comes with potatoes or rice, ask for a substitute of extra vegetables or a side salad.

- Dress your salads with vinaigrette, lemon juice, or olive oil and vinegar. Avoid other dressings.

- Your needs are important so take the time to sit down at a restaurant that serves good quality, nutritious meals. Commit to budget at least twenty minutes for lunch each workday. Even getting into your car and driving to a fast food restaurant takes time. Take a few more minutes to enjoy a sit-down lunch. It just takes intention, follow-through, and a sense of worthiness.

- When your meal arrives, take a few seconds to notice the colors and aroma of your food. Feel grateful for the luxury of having a meal served to you. Turn off your cell phone, and eat slowly. Enjoy your meal in silence by yourself or in quiet conversation with people whose company you enjoy. Leave out conversation, either mentally or out loud, that will provoke anxiety, tension, or stress. Choose your restaurant partners intentionally. Eat mindfully and truly enjoy your food.

AFFIRMATIONS FOR
WEIGHT LOSS AT RESTAURANTS

"I deserve some quiet time each day to enjoy a nutritious meal."

"I'm finding it easier and easier to ignore fast foods."

"I enjoy the habit of eating healthy meals at restaurants."

*"My body needs me as its advocate. I can ask for
healthy choices at restaurants."*

*"I choose to spend my money at restaurants that cater
to health-conscious patrons."*

"My eyes wander effortlessly to the healthy entrée menu choices."

SUCCESS JOURNAL ENTRY

*Describe how often you eat out—either in your hometown—
or when traveling for business or pleasure. What is your
normal fare when you do eat out? Do you often consume refined
carbohydrates, alcohol, fried foods, and desserts?*

*Now list what choices you will make in the future.
Treat this as a grand adventure where you can truly enjoy
eating out and still be true to your health plan.*

Describe your normal restaurant experience up until now.

_____

_____

_____

_____

_____

_____

*Now, list how you will dine out in the future, which restaurants you
will choose, how you will eat mindfully, healthily, and joyfully.
Make these your new affirmations.*

_____

_____

_____

_____

_____

_____

Bon Appetit!

— A FINAL NOTE FROM THE AUTHOR —

Writing this book and being a partner in your weight loss journey has been a true pleasure. You can feel proud for loving yourself and for giving yourself permission to create the good health, slender body, and happiness you deserve. Remember to speak to yourself with kindness, patience, and respect and to treat your body as your best friend. I wish you well as you continue on your success path as the fit and healthy person you were born to be.

Feel free to write to me with your success stories and insights. I would love to hear from you! I can be reached at:

Kristin@newhealthvisions.com or by visiting my website
www.newhealthvisions.com.

— APPENDIX A: RECOMMENDED RESOURCES —

- New Health Visions LLC Hypnosis Recordings
www.NewHealthVisions.com

- *Evolve Your Brain,* Dispenza, Joe, D.C.
Health Communications Inc., 2007

- *UltraMetabolism*, Hyman, Mark, M.D., Atria Books, 2006

- *The UltraSimple Diet*, Hyman, Mark, M.D., Pocket Books, 2007

- *The Rosedale Diet*, Rosedale, Ron, M.D., Harper Collins, 2004

- *The Skinny on Losing Weight without Being Hungry*,
Aronne, Louis, M.D., Broadway Books, 2009

- *Eat This, Not That!*, Zinczenko, David, Rodale Books, 2007

- *Master Your Metabolism*, Michaels, Jillian, Crown Publishers, 2009

- Mercola.com, articles and products, Mercola, Joseph, D.O.

- *The China Study*, Campbell, Collin T, Ph.D. and
Campbell, Thomas M., Benbella Books, 2006

- *Fast Track One-Day Detox Diet*, Gittleman, Ann Louise,
Morgan Road Books, 2005

- *The Detox Strategy*, Watson, Brenda, C.N.C.
with Smith, Leonard, M.D., Free Press, 2008

- *Timeless Healing*, Benson, Herbert, M.D., Simon & Schuster, 1997

- *The Power Of The Mind To Heal*, Borysenko, Joan, Ph.D.,
and Boryseko, Miroslav, Ph.D., Hay House, Inc., 1994

- *You Can Heal Your Life*, Hay, Louise, Hay House, 1999

- *The Power of Intention*, Dyer, Wayne, Ph.D., Hay House, 2005

- *Superfoods*, Wolfe, David, North Atlantic Books, 2009

— APPENDIX B: LEARN MORE ABOUT HYPNOSIS —

In 1958 the American Medical Association formally approved hyp-nosis as a medical tool. According to an article published in *American Health* (September 1986), "Trance Your Self into Better Habits," hyp-nosis has gone mainstream. In this same article, Stanford psychiatrist David Spiegel is quoted as saying:

> *Hypnotizable people can narrow the focus of their attention by turning down the noise in their minds. That's why hypnosis works so well for habit control. It helps people concentrate on a strategy for change without a lot of distracting or negative thoughts.*

Indeed, results of a study showed that when weight loss programs added hypnosis to the treatment plan, weight loss increased by an average of 97 percent. Results were even more spectacular after the program ended. The addition of hypnosis was found to increase weight loss over time by 146 percent (*Journal of Consulting and Clinical Psychology*, 1996)!

Even though hypnosis has been used for decades in the fields of medicine, psychiatry, psychology, and sports it remains a source of un-warranted controversy, skepticism, and fear. This is mainly because stage hypnosis and Hollywood movies have given the impression that the hypnotist takes control of a subject's mind and then has complete power over them. Although this is great for Vegas shows and the movie industry, it has caused people to fear all hypnosis, including ethically practiced clinical hypnotherapy.

The truth is that stage hypnotists select only those people in the audience who want to participate and who show the most suggest-ibility. I have met many people who said they participated at a Vegas show and loved being on stage. They enjoyed feeling uninhibited and the center of attention. In fact, my first Yellow Page ad representative told me that he had a wonderful time at a hypnosis show. A very quiet and conservatively dressed man, he related that he volunteered to go on stage and followed the hypnotist's instructions to relax. With a laugh, he told me that at one point, he was instructed to see everyone in the audience naked! He said that although he knew it wasn't really true, his imagination took over and allowed him this image. "It was really fun, and I was aware of everything," he said.

In reality, hypnosis is a natural state of mind that we routinely enter and exit several times each day—while reading a book, listening to music, watching TV, daydreaming—even while driving a car! Each individual has the power and ability to move in or out of hypnosis at will once they understand what it is and how it is achieved.

Hypnotic suggestion from a trained and experienced practitioner, along with the power of your own concentration and determination, can help you realize many of the life goals that may have once seemed so elusive. The truth is that no one can hypnotize you without your permission and willing participation. No one takes control of your mind. In fact, quite the opposite is true: *hypnosis gives you back control, allowing you self-mastery, empowerment, and confidence.*

■ *HOW DOES HYPNOSIS WORK?*

Having an undesirable habit that we want to stop, but find virtually impossible to do so, is not a matter of personal weakness or a lack of willpower. It can be seen as a function of how our minds work: the two parts of our mind, our *conscious mind* and our *subconscious mind*, are often in conflict. In general, the conscious mind is involved in problem solving. It is our awareness and represents what we commonly refer to as "willpower." Conversely, although the subconscious mind is very powerful and protective of you, it lacks the thinking and rationalizing abilities of the conscious mind. It is more like a computer, with a massive database that stores memories of events and emotions. It is also where our habits are formed and kept.

Under hypnosis, the subconscious mind becomes accessible and open to suggestions that you want to hear. It then stores this new information about the changes you want to make. When the conscious and subconscious minds view a problem (or habit) similarly, changes can be surprisingly easy to make.

Consider this: It is commonly agreed that the conscious mind is only 10 percent of our total mind, with the subconscious mind making up the remaining 90 percent. As I tell my clients, especially those who desperately want to quit smoking but are fearful of failing: "Your conscious mind, knowing all of the reasons why smoking is so damaging, motivated you to come here, but your subconscious mind is yelling 'no!' "

This is because the subconscious mind is still programmed with positive, albeit faulty and irrational, associations with smoking. Hypnosis opens the door between the two minds, allowing the truth about cigarettes to flow unimpeded into the subconscious mind.

Once people recognize that bad habits are not their fault, but are simply a matter of faulty programming, the guilt, shame, and fear of failure is lifted and healing can begin.

This works identically well with all habits that we wish to change. Once the two minds are in sync, change can be effortless, quick, and permanent. In other words, once your subconscious mind is programmed with the truth about food: that it is not your friend, reward, or entertainment, but is only a source for good quality physical nourishment, emotional eating can cease once and for all.

■ WHAT DOES HYPNOSIS FEEL LIKE?

While in a state of hypnosis, your breathing slows, your heartbeat decreases, and the muscles in your body become completely relaxed. Mentally and physically, it is an extremely pleasant sensation. Some people experience a feeling of lightness; others feel a wonderful sense of heaviness in their limbs. Because you remain mentally alert and because it is not a new experience, some may even doubt that they were hypnotized. A look at the clock will usually dispel this notion. Most people think they "were under" for only five to ten minutes, but are amazed to see their hypnosis session was actually forty minutes or longer!

■ *IS HYPNOSIS SAFE?*

As a naturally occurring event, the hypnotic state is perfectly safe. One of the most common fears surrounding hypnosis is the fear of losing control. Actually, you cannot be hypnotized unless you want to be hypnotized. And because you will never lose consciousness and will hear every word during your session, you will never relinquish control of your own self-will and decision-making abilities.

If a suggestion were made that you fundamentally disagreed with or resented, you would simply emerge from this state of relaxation on your own. This is why it is so important for you and your hypnotherapist to understand and agree on your goals before hypnotic induction. Your choice of hypnotherapist should be a well-trained professional whom you can trust to work with you.

I can't tell you how many times a new client has nervously asked, "You won't make me quack like a duck, will you?" I smile and joke, "You don't need hypnosis for that. You can quack like a duck any time you want. Let's work on something more challenging."

Of course, they are referring to the common fear of a post-hypnotic suggestion being implanted that will render them duck-like at inappropriate times. But I always take the time to explain that they can never be made to do anything they do not want to do. In fact, the time I take during a first session where I discuss the truth about hypnosis, what it feels like, and how it works is just as important as the hypnosis itself.

■ *HOW DO I KNOW I CAN BE HYPNOTIZED?*

Virtually anyone who wants to be hypnotized can be hypnotized! There are three basic factors that will influence your success with hypnosis:
- Your willingness to be hypnotized
- How effectively you use your imagination
- Your motivation to accomplish your goals

The clinical hypnotherapist is merely a guide who will gently lead and assist you into your relaxed state.

■ *HOW CAN HYPNOSIS HELP ME?*

With the help of a trained and skilled hypnotherapist, hypnosis is a safe, yet powerful, method to help in many ways to:

- Lose weight
- Stop smoking
- Ease or even completely release pain
- Reduce or eliminate stress
- Increase motivation
- Enhance learning
- Increase concentration
- Reduce or eliminate fears
- Stop addictions
- Stop nail biting
- Improve sports performance
- Eliminate fear of public speaking
- Get rid of stage fright
- Lower blood pressure
- Reduce or eliminate dental anxiety
- Improve mental health
- Increase creativity
- Reduce or eliminate anxiety
- Improve self-esteem
- Stop procrastination
- End stuttering

■ *QUITTING SMOKING WITH HYPNOSIS*

It is not unusual for my clients to completely quit smoking with just one session. Here's Gail's story, which she asked me to share. Like most people who have smoked for several years, Gail desperately needed to quit but was reluctant to give up her "best friend." Like most people, she was terrified of the withdrawal symptoms, weight gain, moodiness, and sluggishness she always experienced after trying to quit "on her own."

I took my time educating Gail on the basics of clinical hypnosis, and she was able to relax deeply and accept the life-affirming suggestions of being a nonsmoker. She felt wonderful as she left my office saying "I hope I feel this way forever!" Gail has kept in touch with me and is still excited about how beautifully her life has changed since that one session. She recently told me:

I can't believe the energy I now have, starting in the morning and lasting all day. Everyone is noticing it and telling me that I absolutely glow! It's so weird and unbelievable that I don't even want a cigarette when I'm with my smoking friends.

■ SPORTS PERFORMANCE AND HYPNOSIS

Here is the story from my fourteen-year-old client, Ashley:

I was pitching in a softball game when a line drive hit my head, knocking me out. After four weeks on the bench with a bad concussion, I was finally cleared to play. But I was shocked to find out that I was now deathly afraid of the softball, and I mean deathly! I came home from every practice crying, wanting to quit.

When my dad suggested I see a hypnotherapist, my mom found Kristin. Right after my hypnosis session, my fear of the softball was completely gone. I wasn't scared anymore! I could catch anything. I was unstoppable. I would always repeat to myself "I am safe. I am protected," and it worked. Now at every game I'm the player I used to be. I'm an all-star pitcher and still feel unstoppable. If we hadn't seen Kristin, I wouldn't be where I am today. I would still be afraid, and I would never be able to pitch again.

■ END STUTTERING WITH HYPNOSIS

One of the most surprising and even shocking examples of the healing power of the subconscious mind is demonstrated when I use hypnosis to help ease stuttering. In just the past month, I worked with two middle-aged men who developed a sudden and severe case of stuttering following a health crisis. When their medical teams were unable to determine the physical cause and treatment of this issue, they were faced with fear and anguish. Both men were so debilitated by the stuttering that they were barely able to communicate and terrified that they would never regain normal speech again. They were desperate to try anything.

In both cases, the stuttering was eased by at least 98 percent, after just one hypnosis session. As one of the men, Jack, told me:

When I left your office, I was so happy that I could talk again that I couldn't stop talking out loud! I talked and talked in the parking lot and all the way driving home. I just couldn't believe it and was so happy! My doctor and speech therapist almost fell off their chairs when they heard me speak for the first time after my session with you, Kristin. They are now believers in hypnosis, as am I!

■ WEIGHT LOSS SUCCESS WITH HYPNOSIS

My client, David, has a story of weight loss success using hypnosis that is a common one. David had a very stressful sales job at a company that was in deep financial trouble. As the workload and stress increased, David's appetite for fast food, pop, and candy soared. Evenings were the worst, as he found himself giving in to the urge to eat huge, carbohydrate-laden dinners and to snack on chips and cookies all evening. No matter how hard he tried, he just couldn't stop the eating habits that were making him morbidly obese.

With just one session, David was able to turn these habits around and lost six pounds in the first week. At his follow-up session the next week, David said, "I think I have finally found something that will work for me. Food wasn't on my mind 24-7, and I actually wanted to exercise every morning." Like everyone, David feared that this was too good to last. But after several follow-up hypnosis sessions and using my *Hypnosis for Weight Loss* CD daily, David was able to shed and keep off fifty pounds.

A note worth mentioning: Although most habits can be totally eliminated within one to three sessions, weight loss may take a few more sessions, depending on the amount of weight needed to be lost and the underlying emotional issues involved. Using my *Hypnosis for Weight Loss* CD as often as possible remarkably speeds up the process, as it keeps the new mental programming strong and acts as a stress reliever. Instead of eating for relaxation, my clients love to let go of the day's stress by enjoying an at-home hypnosis session. These anecdotal results are backed up by studies that have shown that late night eating is related to an increased level of the stress hormone called cortisol. By using relaxation techniques, thus lowering their cortisol levels, people were able to eliminate this night eating syndrome after just one week.

I invite you to further explore the wonderful ways hypnosis can help you achieve your health goals. Please feel free to visit my interactive website at www.newhealthvisions.com for more information and support.

— ACKNOWLEDGMENTS —

My deep and heartfelt gratitude goes to the following people who helped to inspire and create this book:

To my clients, thank you for placing your trust and faith in my work and for urging me to put my thoughts and techniques in writing. This book would not exist without you.

Loving thanks to Geri Rudd, who taught me the art of hypnotherapy and encouraged me to make it my life's profession.

To Tina Feigal, Montana Gray, and Mary Stoffel, thank you for your editing skills, motivation, and inspiration.

A big thank you to Beaver's Pond Press, especially Dara Beevas, for your mentorship and for sharing in my vision.

To Carol Logie, thank you for the beautiful cover and interior design.

To my many friends who have supported me on this journey, especially Amelia Amon, Elizabeth Bowden, Dee Cantalice, Mike Dooley, Dawn Mathers, Kris Nelson, Maureen Neumann, Karen Rajtar, and Toni Wood. My life is truly enriched by your presence.

To my amazing siblings, my built-in support group, for giving me many lifetimes worth of kindness and love. I treasure each of you. I extend special thanks and gratitude to my brother Tyler Volk, who has paved the way for me in so many areas of life. Thank you for the long phone calls during which you generously dispensed priceless advice and encouragement, and for contributing the title of this book. And to my sister Janice Volk, thank you for not only being an incredible sister but also for being a dear friend. Your companionship and selfless love mean so much to me.

To my husband, Bernard Funk, red pen always at the ready, for patiently reading and editing my manuscript from cover to cover so many times that I lost count, for your valuable literary advice and insights, and for your love and support.

To Ben Volk and Pat Bowers for always cheering me on!

To my late grandparents, Joseph Volk, Angela Volk, and Lucille Ziolek Hellmers, for showing me how to age with grace, wisdom, and beauty.

And, most importantly, to my parents, Vivian Volk, and the late Joseph Volk who always believed in me and whose legacy continues to inspire me everyday.